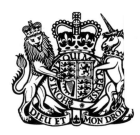

Chronic Disease Management Registers

Proceedings of a Workshop

**Edited and Organised by
Dr Ann Dawson**

Co-Edited by Mark Ferrero

London: HMSO

ISBN 011 321 984 9

Contents

Foreword

Over the past few years there has been a great deal of interest in the use of registers for the management of chronic diseases such as diabetes and asthma, in particular as a means of improving the quality of care delivered. The NHS Executive recognised the potential usefulness of chronic disease management registers in its Chronic Disease Management Programme (CDMP), which requires participating general practices to keep and maintain an up-to-date register of all people with diabetes and/or asthma. Over 95% of general practices receive a special payment for running a CDMP. Several diabetologists have also set up registers of patients attending their outpatient clinics and a few also collect data from local general practices. In addition a few district health authorities have or are in the process of setting up district population-based management registers.

The NHS Executive is not convinced that there is a case for *national* chronic disease management registers. Such national registers are unlikely to add significantly to the quality of individual patient care nor be worth the cost of maintaining and keeping them up to date. We do however believe that district population-based disease management registers may be useful in providing information for the planning and provision of local services. It is for health authorities to decide whether they wish to make the necessary investment to establish and maintain such registers, and to determine the location of the register.

District health authorities which do set up district registers are responsible for the use of the data contained in them, and local arrangements should make this clear. The security and confidentiality of patient data must be protected. Departmental policy on the protection and use of such data is set out in HSG(96)18.

This workshop was specially designed to bring together key people who have set up registers and whose experience would be valuable to other health care planners who are considering following suit. I am very grateful to them for sharing that experience.

Although primarily aimed at colleagues working in health authorities the record of proceedings will also be of value to general practitioners.

Dr Graham Winyard
Medical Director
NHS Executive

Preface

Many health professionals, health service planners and managers, have concluded that population-based disease-specific patient registers are an important component in local service provision for the management of chronic conditions. Research evidence to support this view may not have been systematically reviewed. Nevertheless, it is easy to see that having a basic means of calling and recalling patients for check-ups, coupled with the capacity to record simple information about the progress and management of their illnesses, is likely to lead to a more efficient and effective service, and to provide a valuable source of data to inform future service development and evaluation. The advent of the Chronic Disease Management Programme (CDMP) for the primary care management of diabetes and asthma, signalled an acceptance of the principle of disease-specific patient registers at general practice level, with anonymised data returns being made to the local Family Health Services Authority. Enthusiastic hospital specialists, particularly in the diabetes field, consider that the CDMP registers are too basic, and that more highly-developed, computerised registers are the only way to maximise the benefit both to their patients and to their research. Schools of thought differ as to the precise type of register needed, and where it should be located, and experts continue to debate the subject. Some would even like to see a national diabetes register, although the NHS Executive remains unconvinced by such arguments.

We nonetheless recognised a need to draw together the various strands of the debate and present the key issues in a single reference document, as an aid to health authorities who might be contemplating setting up a disease management register. The detail of local service structure in this area is, of course, a matter for health authorities to determine, in discussion with local interested parties. But there are certain generic legal and operational issues which need to be considered, and certain ground rules to be observed in this process. Data relating to specific patients are clearly sensitive, and the underlying principles of the Data Protection Act and similar legal and ethical duties are well known to health authorities and clinicians alike. Patient data, whether anonymised or not can be a powerful tool to commercial and lobbying interests. Arrangements for gathering, aggregating, storing and using NHS data should be robust enough to ensure, not only that health authorities are able to fulfil their legal responsibilities for the security of such data, but also that no commercial or lobbying interest can exert undue influence over the priorities and structures of local NHS services, nor use data for a purpose that has not been authorised.

The papers included in these proceedings are based on presentations made by the authors at an NHS Executive workshop held in July 1995. Some of the presentations were made by NHS Executive officials, but most were from individuals involved in some aspect of health care with wide experience of setting up registers. With the exception of the NHS Executive papers, the views expressed are those of the authors, and do not necessarily represent NHS Executive policy. However, we thought it would be helpful to introduce each section with an NHS Executive perspective, which can be readily distinguished from the main text. In particular the Department of Health's guidance on the protection and use of patient information was published some time after the workshop and has general applicability.

Finally colleagues will note that as from 1 April 1996 FHSAs and district health authorities referred to throughout these proceedings were merged into unified health authorities.

Dr Ann Dawson
Mark Ferrero

Acknowledgements

Grateful acknowledgement is hereby made to all those professional colleagues who gave their time to participate actively in this workshop and thus generously shared their knowledge. Particular thanks go to Dr Barry Tennison for chairing the workshop, especially for keeping the discussion focussed, and to NHS Executive administrative colleagues Alan Bell, Ann Barker and Simon Claydon for their invaluable help in arranging the workshop, and to Daphne Johnson for secretarial support.

Editor's Note

DiabCare DiabCare

Through out these proceedings reference is made to the WHO EURO diabetes managed care programme. It is either referred to as DiabCare or DiabCare.

We have been advised by WHO EURO and in particular colleagues in the St Vincent Secretariat the both forms of the word heve been used by them in the past, DiabCare being the older form.

Opening Remarks by Chairman

Dr Barry Tennison, Director of Public Health, Hertfordshire Health Agency

I would like to open the day by welcoming you to this workshop and thanking you on behalf of the NHS Executive, for agreeing so readily to participate. Having had an opportunity to review the agenda, I shall be listening with interest to the presentations about existing registers, with the following four connected questions in mind.

1   What is the **definition** of the register: That is, if it worked perfectly, who should (at any particular moment) be on the register, and who should be off?

- Does this depend on a person's address, or on contact with services (where they get treated)?
- What are the criteria (if any) in terms of diagnosis, type of treatment, age?

Is this definition clear and appropriate (for the purposes of the register)?

2   What are the **mechanisms** for keeping the register accurate, complete and up to date?

- How are people put on it and taken off it?
- How is it ensured that all those, and only those, satisfying the definition (1) are there?
- How are changes of name, address or contact with services dealt with?
- What stops the register silting up with undetected duplicates and people who are dead or have moved?

Are these mechanisms adequate for the definition and purposes of the register? Will they actually happen?

3   What are the **purposes** of the register?

- Is it primarily operational, or for monitoring a service, or for epidemiology?
- Do multiple intended purposes conflict too much?

Are the definition and the updating mechanisms sufficient for the register to fulfil its purposes?

4   Are the **practical arrangements** for the register adequate to achieve (1)–(3)?

- Is the information technology appropriate and adequate?
- Are the people actually running it able (and willing) to do so properly?

- Are the paper or other flows and processes well designed?
- Is the register kept in the right place and by the right organisation?

Will it actually work?

You may gather that I start from a somewhat sceptical position, having seen many attempts at registers (of various sorts) which were doomed not to work because those involved thought the problem simple, when in fact it is quite complex.

For example, complexities around these questions include:

1 All diabetics? Type I/II? Treated or not? Transient (eg gestational) included or not?

Geographically (residence) or treatment based? For example, many talk of a "District diabetic register": what does this mean, in terms of intended coverage?

2 Need managerial mechanisms to detect:

- changes of name, address, treatment location (if relevant to definition)
- duplicates, removal of those with later detected misdiagnosis
- death
- significant other events (visual problems, renal problems, cardiovascular disease) if the purpose of the register includes monitoring or surveying these

They need to be realistic in terms of turnaround time and organisational behaviour.

3 Design for an operational system is different from that for an epidemiology or monitoring system. Many claim that a register can monitor outcomes without thinking through what would be necessary to do this (especially in the long term).

4 Experience of FHSAs reveals the frustration of trying to use an operational register for analysis and reporting. Staff need to have an investment in the accuracy and completeness of the register for it to have a chance.

These are my prelminary thoughts which doubtless will be modified once I have hear your presentations.

1
General
Considerations

Overview

In this section, the asthma and diabetes registers which GP practices participating in the Chronic Disease Management Programme (CDMP) are required to keep are explained. Although simple, the case is made that the CDMP registers are the obvious place to start if contemplating the establishment of a district population-based register. Data from registers can be used for monitoring health outcomes, and a series of case studies are used to highlight ways in which this might be done. The status quo of district population-based registers is reviewed and the wider implications for health authorities contemplating setting up such a register are explored, including the economic issues. The key message emerging is that the rules governing the protection and use of patient data are crucial. The Department of Health has recently published guidance on this point [Ref HSG (96) 18]. Purchasing health authorities are the logical location for a district population-based register as they are the guardians of NHS paper and computer data and have a central role in identifying health needs of local populations, planning to meet these needs and in monitoring both health outcomes and the quality and effectiveness of local health services.

1.1 Registers and Chronic Disease Management

Mark Ferrero, Principal Administrator, Health Care Directorate,
NHS Executive, London

Introduction

The Chronic Disease Management Programme (CDMP) came about as a result of the growth of health promotion clinics—mostly for asthma and diabetes—in primary care. GPs were paid if they ran such clinics, but there were wide variations in what was provided. In order to provide a framework for the clinics, a separate programme was launched in July 1993—the Chronic Disease Management Programme. Well over 90% GP of practices now take part in the CDMP, and consequently there is already a lot of data in GP surgeries.

CDMPs for Asthma and Diabetes

The CDMPs for diabetes and asthma have a lot in common with each other. Among their common features are requirements:-

i)   To keep registers of patients suffering from either disease;

ii)   To ensure systematic call and recall of patients takes place, either in hospital or primary care;

iii) To carry out regular reviews, including tests and checks (peak-flow, complications): six–monthly for asthma; annually for diabetes;

iv)   To keep records of the procedures required under the programme, incorporating information from other providers involved (eg hospitals, community units);

v)   To carry out clinical audit.

Report to the FHSA

In addition to the procedures required at practice level, the Family Health Services Authority (FHSA) requires an annual report covering:–

i)   For asthma:–
      • the number of asthma patients distributed by age and sex;
      • the number of asthma patients who have:

      a) received regular prophylactic medication;

b) had peak flow measurement in the past year;

c) been admitted to hospital.

ii)   For diabetes:–

- the number of diabetes patients who are insulin dependent
- the number of diabetes patients who are non–insulin dependent
- the number of diabetes patients who have had a follow-up review (including checks for complications) in:

    a) a hospital or shared care programme; and

    b) the practice alone.

What the CDMP does not Stipulate

With regard to information storage and retrieval, there are two important aspect the CDMP does not prescribe:

i)   how the information should be stored; and

i)   how information from other providers is to be obtained legitimately for incorporation.

The way in which information collected under the CDMP is stored will vary from practice to practice—electronic databases will occur in computerised practises, others may have a card index or other non-electronic methods.

Procedures for exchanging information across the primary/secondary care interface will vary—in both type and reliability. In some areas there may be registers in GP practices existing alongside a register in the local hospital or diabetes centre. Information in these registers will inevitably overlap, but neither will be complete. 'Duplicate' entries will abound, as well as 'ghosts', that is, people who have moved away or died and not been deleted from the register.

Why are CDMP Registers Needed?

CDMP registers are a vital information resource to the general practice and the FHSA.

CDMP registers can help reduce the adverse effects of the diseases by enabling primary care teams to:–

i)   monitor more effectively all patients who have been diagnosed as having either diabetes or asthma and to detect at an early stage those whose condition is worsening or who are developing complications;

ii)   empower patients by ensuring they, and their families or carers, receive the necessary education in the nature of the disease and how they can take maximum responsibility for its management;

iii)   call and recall patients effectively for health checks and continuing education;

iv)   identify as early as possible those patients likely need the care of a specialist (eg chest consultant) or other care professionals (eg chiropodist, surgeon) and refer them on promptly.

CDMP registers also:–

i)   enable clinical audit to be carried out to determine the effectiveness of interventions and disease management; and

iii)   provide epidemiological data to build a local picture at FHSA level.

Shortcomings of CDMP Registers

There is no doubt that the information contained in CDMP registers is important and useful, but:–
- it is basic;
- it is stored differently from practice to practice;
- its accessibility, potential for easy analysis, and reliability are all variable;
- it cannot easily be aggregated for more detailed epidemiological analysis; and
- it cannot easily be enhanced without adding to the paperwork in doctors' practices.

Key questions

A number of questions about CDMP registers need to be raised in any wider consideration of registers. These are:–

i)   Should GPs be encouraged to record information over and above what is required under the CDMP? How might this be achieved? What does the GP stand to gain?

ii)   What essential additional information should be recorded, and why?

iii)   What is the role of hospital-based registers? Are they necessary as well as CDMP registers?

iv)   How can hospitals work more effectively with primary care to capitalise on the information held in the CDMP registers?

v)   How can patients themselves, and their carers, take greater responsibility for the accuracy and completeness of information about them held on registers?

Conclusion

CDMP registers are an important feature in the effective management of chronic diseases in primary care. They contain much useful information for other purposes, and despite their shortcomings, CDMP registers offer terrific potential. The key issue is how to harness the information they contain and maximise their potential.

Reference

1 Statement of Fees and Allowances (The Red Book). (1990), para 30 et seq, schedules 4 & 5. *The Chronic Disease Management Programme*

1.2   Use of Data from Registers for Monitoring Outcomes

Dr Azim Lakhani, Director, Central Health Outcomes Unit, Department of Health, London

Introduction

"To secure through the resources available, the greatest improvement in the physical and mental health of people in England"

This statement of goals has been with the NHS in one form or another ever since its inception. Most people associated with the NHS share this goal and wish to contribute to its achievement while acknowledging that health is influenced by wider efforts of society as well as by health care. This, therefore, forms a useful basis for defining the end points of health interventions and exploring the role of outcomes assessment in improving their delivery. This paper attempts to use several case studies to illustrate this role. The paper also highlights current constraints with such assessment in the NHS which need resolving to make its contribution a reality and the potential role of information from registers.

Key Questions and Issues

There is a belief that clinical care is of the highest quality and offers optimal benefit. The NHS must now be able *to demonstrate* this, not just make claims about it.

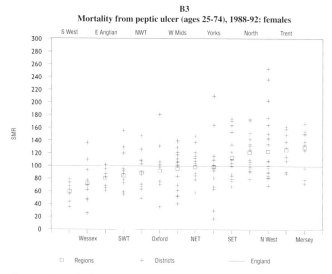

B3
Mortality from peptic ulcer (ages 25-74), 1988-92: females

Source - Population Health Outcome Indicators for the NHS 1993

Case Study 1 (Department of Health 1993, Lakhani 1993) shows data on deaths due to peptic ulcers, standardised for age and sex, by district and regional health authority in England. There is marked variation in mortality which is considered potentially preventable for the age groups stated. This is typical of variation in clinical practice, resource use and outcomes seen repeatedly, whether based on routine data, audit or rigorous research. It is such variation that raises questions about the extent to which the NHS' health goal is being achieved. There may well be valid reasons for some of the death rates as shown in the model in **case study 1** and the reasons may

ACTION FOR HEALTH - PEPTIC ULCER: CASE STUDY 1

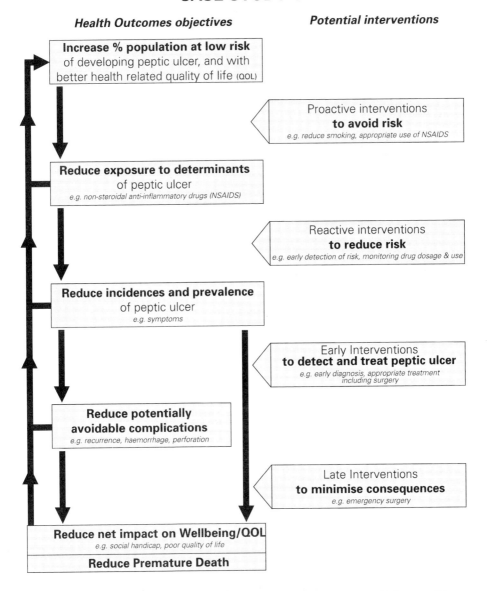

Health Outcomes objectives   *Potential interventions*

Increase % population at low risk of developing peptic ulcer, and with better health related quality of life (QOL)

Proactive interventions **to avoid risk** *e.g. reduce smoking, appropriate use of NSAIDS*

Reduce exposure to determinants of peptic ulcer *e.g. non-steroidal anti-inflammatory drugs (NSAIDS)*

Reactive interventions **to reduce risk** *e.g. early detection of risk, monitoring drug dosage & use*

Reduce incidences and prevalence of peptic ulcer *e.g. symptoms*

Early Interventions **to detect and treat peptic ulcer** *e.g. early diagnosis, appropriate treatment including surgery*

Reduce potentially avoidable complications *e.g. recurrence, haemorrhage, perforation*

Late Interventions **to minimise consequences** *e.g. emergency surgery*

Reduce net impact on Wellbeing/QOL *e.g. social handicap, poor quality of life*

Reduce Premature Death

Central Health Outcomes Unit
Department of Health September 1995

vary from district to district. They need further local investigation and explanation. In some cases the death rates may reflect quality of care. Most of the data required for the model in **case study 1** is not currently available from routine data sets.

Key issues thus are:
- how can the NHS define and demonstrate the outcome of clinical care?
- how can the NHS use information on outcomes to improve care?

The ultimate goal is to achieve the greatest potential benefit, in terms of improved health, from available resources. Having said this, the technical difficulties involved are acknowledged. However, these should be considered *challenges, not an excuse* for not examining outcomes. The following section presents a series of questions the NHS might ask about outcomes, and issues raised by such questions.

What is the Health Problem?

The first question facing the NHS is to understand the clinical and health problems presented by patients and the population. It is becoming increasingly necessary now to extend the scope of this beyond just the clinical features of the problem. For example, **case study 2** on stroke, shows that it is not just pathology, clinical symptoms and signs and death rates that matter. Clinicians are increasingly being required to consider wider aspects such as disability and handicap caused by a clinical disorder; how the patients are able to function; and how they feel about their situation and its impact on the quality of their life and the lives of their families and carers. For patients with stroke and their carers, it is often the latter that are of most concern. Surely it is such broader concerns that should shape the information and data collection agenda. The clinician also needs to consider the *severity* of the presenting problem and its *causes*. In many cases the causes of the presenting problem may be preventable, and the presenting problem itself may represent a negative outcome of previous care or lack of care.

Case Study 2 shows for example, that there is a rising trend in obesity, which is likely to lead to a higher population distribution of blood pressure. A significant proportion of the population still remains with untreated high blood pressure. In defining the health problems, the incidence of stroke and its consequences can not be isolated from trends in high blood pressure and its determinants. The kinds of data shown on the left hand side of the model in **case study 2** are not currently available from routine data sets but could be derived from special registers.

What can the NHS do about the problem?

The decision on what to do should ideally be based on sound research evidence showing that an intervention is likely to lead to a benefit. The

MONITORING OUTCOMES - STROKE:
ILLUSTRATIVE DATA - CASE STUDY 2

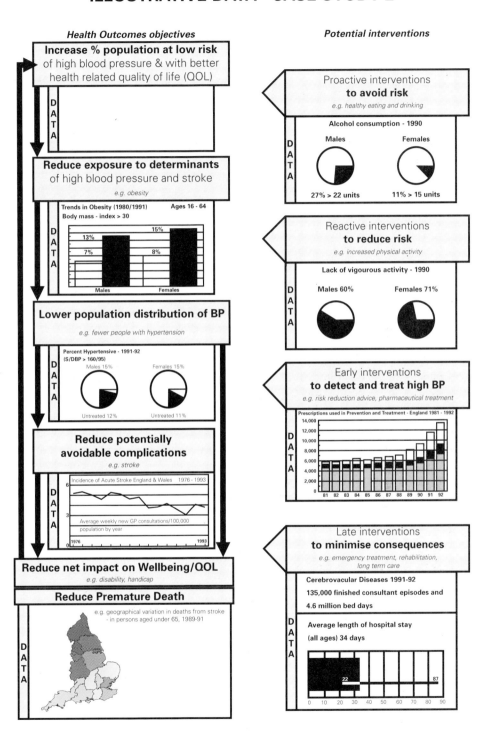

Health Outcomes objectives

Increase % population at low risk
of high blood pressure & with better health related quality of life (QOL)

DATA

Reduce exposure to determinants
of high blood pressure and stroke
e.g. obesity

DATA

Trends in Obesity (1980/1991)   Ages 16 - 64
Body mass - index > 30
15%
13%
7%   8%
Males   Females

Lower population distribution of BP
e.g. fewer people with hypertension

DATA

Percent Hypertensive - 1991-92
(S/DBP > 160/95)
Males 15%   Females 15%
Untreated 12%   Untreated 11%

Reduce potentially avoidable complications
e.g. stroke

DATA

Incidence of Acute Stroke England & Wales   1976 - 1993
Average weekly new GP consultations/100,000
population by year
1976   1993

Reduce net impact on Wellbeing/QOL
e.g. disability, handicap

Reduce Premature Death
e.g. geographical variation in deaths from stroke - in persons aged under 65, 1989-91

DATA

Potential interventions

Proactive interventions
to avoid risk
e.g. healthy eating and drinking

DATA

Alcohol consumption - 1990
Males   Females
27% > 22 units   11% > 15 units

Reactive interventions
to reduce risk
e.g. increased physical activity

DATA

Lack of vigourous activity - 1990
Males 60%   Females 71%

Early interventions
to detect and treat high BP
e.g. risk reduction advice, pharmaceutical treatment

DATA

Prescriptions used in Prevention and Treatment - England 1981 - 1992
14,000
12,000
10,000
8,000
6,000
4,000
2,000
0
81 82 83 84 85 86 87 88 89 90 91 92

Late interventions
to minimise consequences
e.g. emergency treatment, rehabilitation, long term care

DATA

Cerebrovacular Diseases 1991-92
135,000 finished consultant episodes and
4.6 million bed days

Average length of hospital stay
(all ages) 34 days

22   87
0 10 20 30 40 50 60 70 80 90

Source of Data: Various DoH sources

Central Health Outcomes Unit
Department of Health June 1995

scarcity of such research information is well known. An additional concern is that previous research is mostly based on clinical end-points and often does not show effectiveness in terms of well being or impact on quality of life. In the absence of such research evidence, decision making about intervention tends to be based on judgement and peer opinion. Unfortunately, there isn't always agreement on this, which is a key cause of the observed variation in practice and outcomes. It is also widely acknowledged now that individual health professionals can not work in isolation. Most health problems require many professions working together, hence decision making about intervention needs a collaborative approach.

What are the objectives of treatment?

Case Study 3 presents an overview of the range of issues involved in understanding the health problem and making decisions about what to do about asthma. This figure is in two parts:

- The left hand side shows a sequence of events ranging from exposure to causes of asthma, to development of asthma and acute attacks, its complications and consequences such as handicap, poor quality of life and premature death.
- The right hand side shows a whole range of clinical actions aimed at influencing different parts of this sequence.

This raises the next question—what are the objectives of treatment? These will obviously vary with where the patient is within this sequence of events. For example, for someone likely to be exposed to a cause such as pollen in the environment, the objective is to avoid this leading to an asthma attack by prescribing prophylactic drugs. For someone already suffering from an attack, the objective is to detect it early and treat it, to prevent it becoming a prolonged and severe attack.

Whose perspective?

In arriving at a decision about treatment, clinicians need to consider *net* benefit, given that some treatments have side effects and may even cause harm. In considering such *net* benefit, clinicians need to take into account a variety of perspectives and concerns. For example, in the treatment of asthma, the clinician may be more concerned about changes in lung function, the patient more about quality of life, given strict prevention and treatment regimes. The outcomes which patients wish to see changed may include aspects such as sleep disturbance caused by wheeze, having to take time off school and work, feeling isolated at school due to not being able to take part in physical activities etc. This raises key issues about the extent to which patients are involved in decision making about objectives and outcomes. Alongside those of clinicians and patients, the perspectives and values of carers, managers, policy makers, public, researchers and others may also have to be taken into account. Specification of outcomes objectives has implications for data collection.

ACTION FOR HEALTH - ASTHMA: CASE STUDY 3

Health Outcomes objectives

Potential interventions

Increase % population at low risk
of asthma, and with better
health related quality of life (QOL)

Issues
- In the absence of routine measures, use whole population as a proxy

Reduce exposure to determinants
of asthma and acute attacks
e.g. allergens

Issues
- Uncertainty about causes of asthma/attacks
  - Some allergens
  - Maternal smoking
  - Air pollutants
  - Dietary sodium in males
  - Psychosocial problems
  - Viral infection
- Need for research on causes
- Lack of data on incidence and prevalence of causes

Reduce incidence and prevalence
of asthma and acute attacks
e.g. symptoms

Issues
- Lack of local information on incidence and prevalence
- Prevalence range:
  - 3-4% general population
  - 5-15% children
- Lack of agreement on criteria for diagnosis

Reduce potentially
avoidable complications
e.g. severe attacks

Issues
- Confidential enquiries suggest some of these complications are potentially avoidable
- Lack of local data on incidence of complications
- Need for targets for reduction in complications

Reduce net impact on Wellbeing/QOL
e.g. sleepless nights, time of school/work

Reduce Premature Death

Issues
- A study in Southampton (BMJ 1992; 304; 361 - 4) showed:
  - 51% asthma patients waking up at night with wheeze
  - 45% wheezy at least once a week
  - 31% missed school or work in previous year
  - 23% avoided certain physical activities
- Such consequences could be part of audit of outcome
- Such outcomes have implications for non-NHS costs
  e.g. time off work. These costs are not currently known
- Changing trends/geographical variations in death rates
- Some deaths are potentially avoidable - ref. British Thoracic Association Confidential Enquiry

Proactive interventions
to avoid risk
e.g. house cleaning

Issues
- Health professionals need to work with communities on avoiding risks
- NHS costs of avoiding risk are not known
- Non-NHS costs of avoiding risk are not known

Reactive interventions
to reduce risk
e.g. prophylaxis

Issues
- Health professionals need to work with patients and families on information and education about reducing risks
- Variations in prescription rates of preventive drugs
- Appropriateness of balance between prophylaxis and treatment

Early Interventions
to detect and treat asthma
e.g. home peak flow meters, effective drug treatment

Issues
- Rising trend in consultation numbers and rates
- Estimated annual costs of NHS primary and community care in England, including prescriptions - £400 million
- Variations in prescription rates of preventive drugs
- Guidelines on past practice not always followed (EL(93)115)
- Need for integration of primary and secondary care
- Health professionals need to work in alliance with others e.g. school teachers to prevent/recognise severe attacks
- Need to enhance self care

Late Interventions
to minimise consequences
e.g. emergency hospitalisation

Issues
- Estimated annual costs of NHS hospitalisation £40 million
- Variations in hospitalisation
- Confidential enquiries suggest some episodes leading to hospitalisation are potentially avoidable
- Need to audit effectiveness of hospital treatment

Central Health Outcomes Unit
Department of Health September 1995

What are the services required?

Once the objectives are clear, clinicians may be in a position to specify the interventions, services or treatments. In some cases this may involve a single intervention e.g a prescribed pharmaceutical drug, but in many cases this will involve a whole range of interventions over time, involving many professionals working in different parts of the NHS and even outside it. For example, **case study 1** shows an overview of a range of interventions required to manage peptic ulcers and their consequences. The patient may be an active partner in such interventions, particularly so with avoidance of risk and compliance with medication. Alongside data on health, registers would need to have some data on interventions.

What are the standards required?

Achievement of the best possible outcomes may be dependent on delivering services to specified standards. The guidelines on asthma care in EL(93)115 (NHS Management Executive, 1993) attempt to specify such standards.

What are the results?

Once the care is delivered, key questions involve assessing the extent to which the desired results were achieved. The first question is an audit of the quality of service delivery. Was the service delivered to the standards specified? Such information may suggest that the desired benefit is likely to be achieved, hence act as a proxy for future outcome.

Case Study 4 shows how population coverage of screening for cervical cancer may act as a proxy for a future health outcome, avoidance of invasive cervical cancer. This may be supplemented by data from cancer registries, particularly data on cancer stage showing a trend towards earlier stages i.e cancers are being detected early. The second, more important but more difficult question is whether the clinical problems changed as expected, e.g control of asthma symptoms, quality of life (**case study 3**), and whether *this was due* to the clinical action. Such attribution is difficult, as it needs to take into account other possible influences on health and also allow for the presenting problem and its severity. However, without such attribution, the NHS will not be able to demonstrate that it achieved the greatest improvement in health using its resources and action.

This is what we mean by outcome. Once again, this has implications for data collection and data on registers would need to include data on services and interventions.

HON - B2
Incidence of invasive cervical cancer (ICD 180) by RHA and DHA

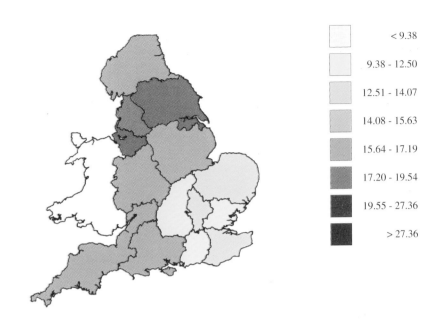

	< 9.38
	9.38 - 12.50
	12.51 - 14.07
	14.08 - 15.63
	15.64 - 17.19
	17.20 - 19.54
	19.55 - 27.36
	> 27.36

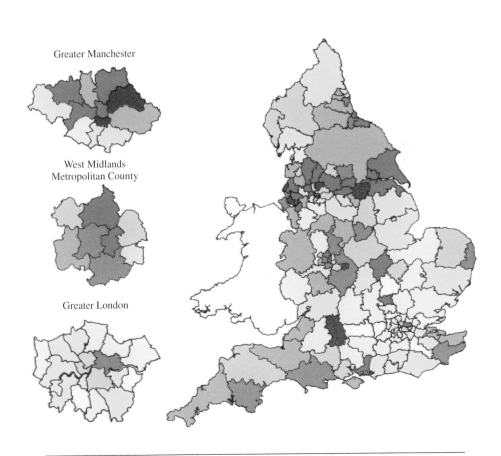

Greater Manchester

West Midlands
Metropolitan County

Greater London

ACTION FOR HEALTH - CERVICAL CANCER:
CASE STUDY 4

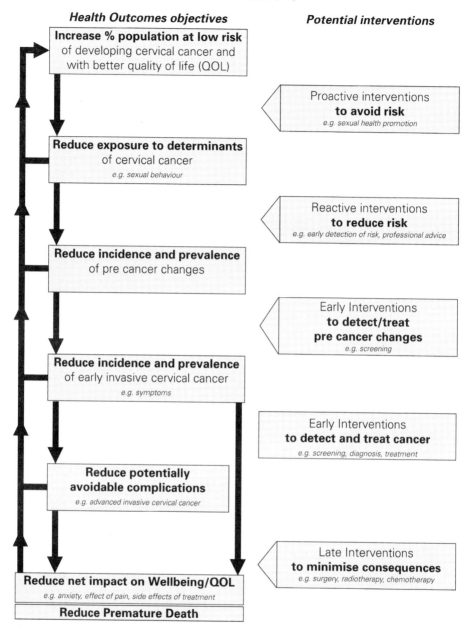

Health Outcomes objectives

Potential interventions

Increase % population at low risk of developing cervical cancer and with better quality of life (QOL)

Proactive interventions **to avoid risk** *e.g. sexual health promotion*

Reduce exposure to determinants of cervical cancer *e.g. sexual behaviour*

Reactive interventions **to reduce risk** *e.g. early detection of risk, professional advice*

Reduce incidence and prevalence of pre cancer changes

Early Interventions **to detect/treat pre cancer changes** *e.g. screening*

Reduce incidence and prevalence of early invasive cervical cancer *e.g. symptoms*

Early Interventions **to detect and treat cancer** *e.g. screening, diagnosis, treatment*

Reduce potentially avoidable complications *e.g. advanced invasive cervical cancer*

Late Interventions **to minimise consequences** *e.g. surgery, radiotherapy, chemotherapy*

Reduce net impact on Wellbeing/QOL *e.g. anxiety, effect of pain, side effects of treatment*

Reduce Premature Death

Central Health Outcomes Unit
Department of Health September 1995

The Department of Health uses this working definition of health outcome (Department of Health 1994):

"Attributable effect of intervention or its lack on a previous health state"

This is still evolving and suggestions for improving on it are most welcome.

Some of the issues in **case study 3** concern variation in population rates for consultation, hospital admissions and deaths due to asthma. Once again, there may well be valid reasons for such variation. However, it does raise questions about the extent to which the NHS is achieving optimum potential benefit from its asthma services, on which it spends some £500 million per annum.

How May Outcomes Assessment be used to Improve Health Intervention and Health?

There are two broad ways in which outcomes measurement may lead to improvements in health interventions and health.
- *promoting* measurement and its use;
- *effecting* use and impact through contracting, advocacy and partnership.

Promoting use

The main responsibility for detailed outcomes assessment and its use lies with the professions. NHS managers and policy makers generally need a broader assessment of outcomes, at a macro level. **Case study 2** (Department of Health 1994) on high blood pressure and stroke care presents a good example of the need to bring a variety of health professionals, different NHS sectors e.g primary and secondary care, and patients together to tackle the issues. The Department of Health is supporting a whole range of projects, working closely with the professions, NHS colleagues and patients to do this. Such joint work engenders a sharing of concerns and issues and ownership of the solutions. These initiatives are described in a leaflet on the work of the Department's Central Health Outcomes Unit (Department of Health 1994). The initiatives will not provide all the answers, methods and systems needed, but will gradually take us forward in our thinking and ability to work with outcomes as part of clinical and NHS care. A significant result of this enormous set of activities on all fronts is that it has stimulated *a more self-questioning culture*, an important stepping stone for today's topic.

Effecting change

The above sections present a theoretical framework of issues. However, unless we are able to apply it to the services in practice we are unlikely to achieve the goals stated earlier. **Case study 2** shows how we might actually use outcomes information to stimulate constructive challenge in order to initiate change in services, leading to better care and, over time, better health. The NHS has 3 broad mechanisms for effecting change:

- a direct mechanism, mostly through management of service provision and contracting for services;
- through advocacy, alerting non–NHS organisations on their contributions to health/ill health and implications for the NHS;
- through partnership with other organisations, even sharing resources to achieve shared and common goals.

Case Study 2 on high blood pressure and stroke illustrates how outcomes assessment may contribute to these, for example, through the NHS:

- highlighting the negative trends in risk of developing high blood pressure e.g obesity, lack of physical activity, and working with other organisations to attempt to reverse them;
- monitoring levels of blood pressure in the population, both to assess outcomes of prevention and treatment initiatives as well as to forecast future incidence of stroke;
- monitoring trends in the incidence of stroke as an indicator of outcome of its high blood pressure prevention and treatment strategies;
- measuring aspects such as function, disability, handicap, well being and, health related quality of life of patients with stroke, and their impact on relatives and carers, as indicators of outcome of stroke treatment, rehabilitation and long term NHS and social care;
- monitoring premature death rates as an indicator of an extreme and potentially avoidable negative outcome of collective NHS and wider influences.

While not all of these measurements are possible at this stage, **case study 2** illustrates that we have enough data at present at national level from sources including special surveys, to question at a macro level, whether the NHS is achieving optimal effectiveness having invested enormous resources annually. Data from registers could enhance this exercise substantially, particularly at local level. Most of the resources used for high blood pressure and stroke are concentrated at the lower end of the chart, on treatment, rehabilitation and long term care following stroke. Such data may be used as part of the strategic planning and contracting process to effect the required changes in service provision to improve outcomes.

Conclusions

In this paper it has only been possible to cover an overview of key issues concerning the role of outcomes assessment in improving health intervention and health, and the potential use of data from registers for such purposes, as follows:–

- Information on outcomes, focused around particular questions, is likely to make an important contribution to decision making at the local level hence overall effectiveness;
- Development of such information requires a systematic and structured approach;
- There is a need for such information and intelligence to extend beyond the clinical arena, into wider areas such as education and the planning and management of services;
- There is a need for collaboration in the development of methods and systems, in order to avoid duplication of effort;
- There is a substantial collaborative development effort already under way between the Department of Health, the NHS, health professionals, patients and others.

References

1 "Population Health Outcome Indicators for the NHS 1993: A Consultation Document." (Institute of Public Health, University of Surrey. Department of Health, 1993)

2 Central Health Outcomes Unit. (Department of Health, 1994)

3 Lakhani, A., "The role of health outcomes assessment in health care commissioning": In—*Best Practice in Health Care Commissioning* (Eds Peel and Sheaff). (Longman, 1993), 2.7, 1–9

4 *EL(93)115*—"Improving Clinical Effectiveness." (NHS Management Executive, Department of Health, 1993)

1.3 District Population-Based Disease Management Registers: Issues for Health Authority Consideration

Dr Ann Dawson, Senior Medical Officer, Health Care Directorate,

NHS Executive, London

Introduction

General practitioners (GPs) have been encouraged to take a population based approach to health care for some time. This theme extends throughout fundholding, total purchasing, commissioning and health promotion. In 1993 the NHS Executive launched the Chronic Diseases Management Programme (CDMP)[1] for diabetes and asthma, which now involves over 95% of general practices. As a requirement of CDMP each practice has to keep a provider register of all its patients with diabetes and/or asthma, and periodically, must send data to the local Family Health Services Authority (FHSA)*. In some areas attempts have been made to aggregate the diabetes data into a district-based register. This paper reviews the progress to date in establishing district population-based registers. It also identifies some of the more important issues for health care planners in making decisions on the desirability or otherwise, of establishing district population-based registers. Although applicable to all chronic diseases it concentrates primarily on diabetes. More detailed information on the practical aspects of registration and CDMP can be found elsewhere in these proceedings.

Background

Within the last decade a great deal of interest has been shown, at national and international level, in the development of disease management programmes as a means of improving the overall standard of care delivered to patients with chronic diseases such as diabetes and asthma. As part of this initiative much attention has been given to patient registers which professional colleagues claim is a prerequisite for improving the quality of health care delivered [2,3,4,5]

Despite the lack of published evidence supporting the hypothesis that registers help to reduce morbidity, entreprenurial clinicians, have set up or are in the processs of setting up provider and district-based registers, which understandably in the circumstances, are disease specific. A great deal of time and effort has been put into their development because they believe

* To district health authority from April 1996

that a registration system which can identify and monitor the health care delivered must have an impact on the overall standard of care and thus on clinical outcomes, a reasonable supposition which the NHS Executive acknowledged in establishing the CDMP.

Potential Uses of Provider and District Population–based Registers

Provider registers can be useful for a variety of reasons which include:
- the identification of patients;
- call and recall of patients;
- monitoring patients' progress and clinical outcomes generally;

and district population-based registers may:
- facilitate the aggregation and analysis of comparable data to i) enable comparisons to be made over time in primary and secondary care and ii) assist health authorities with their strategic planning.

Current National Situation

An increasing number of registers have been, or are being, set up around the country. Those GPs who have been approved to run the CDMPs for diabetes and asthma already have their own provider registers, as have some hospital-based diabetologists. However should a district population-based register be thought necessary provision should be made at district level, to collate data both from the GP registers and the hospital-based registers. Although a few "district population-based registers" have been set up these involve less than 10% of districts, and are distributed patchily across the country, and all but a handful truly reflect the district population.

1 Types and Location of Registers

Over 95% of all general practices have a diabetes register, usually paper although an increasing number are computerised. Some enterprising general practices have joined with other practices in order to aggregate their data[6]. Obviously data from these registers do not reflect the entire district population. Similarly some diabetologists have set up provider registers which record data from patients attending their outpatient's clinic. These registers are located in the hospital, usually in the diabetes centre. However some of these hospital-based registers also record data from local general practices and closely reflect the district population[7]. Some aggregated registers are also located within the FHSA[8] or in the local Medical Audit Advisory Group (MAAG)[9] and record large numbers of patients from both the primary and secondary sectors and thus more closely reflect the district population.

Issues for health authority consideration:

a) **Why have district population-based registers?**
   To enable health care planners within the health authority to develop strategic policies for chronic disease management.

b) **Where should the district population-based registers be located?**
   At present there is no evidence to indicate that one particular location is better than any other. If a register has already been set up in a district and is operating effectively and meets all the health authority requirements, including data security and confidentiality, then the health authority may wish to commission it, rather than set up a new system.

c) **Who is best placed to co-ordinate the setting up of district population-based register should it be perceived necessary?**
   The health authority on behalf of the Secretary of State for Health has overall responsibility for the provision of health care within their district and therefore it is they who are responsible for collecting this type of data should they deem it necessary.

d) **Do health authorities actually have to set up and run the district population-based register themselves?**
   Health authorities need only have registers if they consider them necessary. If a register is thought necessary then they may, if they wish, commission others to set up the district population-based register, collect the data and analyse it on their behalf. However they should ensure that data collected are for the health authority's use only, and cannot be transmitted to a third party without their prior written consent. This is to ensure that data security and confidentiality is maintained at all times. Patients must also be informed that they are on a register, its purpose explained, and their agreement sought to use that data for each particular purpose.

e) **Do registers need to be disease specific?**
   At general practice level it would be impracticable to expect GPs to have specific registers and software for each disease or condition. Similarly health authorities may prefer to have generic registers rather than disease specific registers.

2 Economic Considerations

The financial implications of setting up registers are detailed elsewhere in these proceedings[10].

Issues for health authority consideration:

a) **Is there any evidence that registers are a cost effective way of reducing morbidity?**
There is little or no published evidence to show that registration of patients with chronic diseases improves their clinical outcome. This creates a dilemma for the local health care planners who wish to ensure that they get the "biggest bang for their bucks" and who need to be assured that registers actually achieve a measurable health gain. It is however widely recognised that registers will probably i) improve local arrangements for the provision of care ii) ensure the appropriate levels of provision iii) enable the delivered care to be reviewed at general practice and at health authority levels all of which should improve clinical outcomes.

b) **Who funds the district population-based registers already in place?**
Health authorities have in some instances commissioned a local diabetologist[11], the local MAAG[9] or a private concern[12] to set up and run district population-based registers on their behalf, and funded them accordingly. However most registers have been set up by diabetologists who have a particular interest in registers and who fund and operate them from their own resources.

3 Software

A variety of software is available for use in primary or secondary care, or both. Software developed in the secondary care sector to meet its own particular needs is now being offered on a commercial basis to other interested parties and has thus become an income generator. The Family Health Service Computer Unit (FHSCU) has also developed specific software for a diabetes register as have commercial companies. Clearly, compatability is a key consideration in ensuring district-wide access to data.

Issues for health authority consideration:

a) **Do general practitioners need special software packages?**
General Practitioners who use computers in their practice will be able to use/modify their own software package, thus avoiding the additional expense of a specific software package.

b) **What is the best software package for use at district level?**
No software package is obviously better than any other. Whatever software is chosen should be simple and easy to use, compatible with other software in use within the district and sophisticated enough to collect, aggregate, analyse and update all the district data. There are a number of software packages on the market for this purpose, however many have proved difficult to operate. Before buying a particular

package, it is generally a good idea to take advice from somebody who has used it.

c)   Has the NHS Executive provided any advice on the new technology?
Yes, the NHS Executive has provide the following advice:

*i) the **NHS-wide networking programme**[13] which aims to ensure that, subject to proper safeguards, by 1996, 90% of all NHS organisations will be able to exchange information electronically.*

*ii) General Medical Computer Systems: the **Requirements for Accreditation Version 3 1995/96**[14] was introduced to ensure that the GMP computer systems provide an agreed core functionality and conform to relevant national standards.*

*iii) **Model Practice Policy on Information Security**[15] which provides a policy framework within which Information Technology can be used in the most secure way, given the demands of a busy practice. Thus all reasonable action should be taken to :*

• ensure confidentiality, so that only authorised persons can access the system and not disclose information to anyone who has no right to see;

• maintain the integrity of the data by taking over input, ensuring that all changes are reported and monitored updating data, checking that the correct record is on the screen before updating, learning how the system should be used and keeping up to date with changes which may affect functionality and reporting all apparent errors and ensuring that they are resolved;

• maintain the availabilty of all data by ensuring that all equipment is protected from intruders, that back up are taken regularly at predetermined intervals and that contingency plans are provided for the possible failure or equipment theft and that any such contingency plans are tested and kept up to date.

4   Datasets

It is important to have an agreed standard dataset so that there is a consistent and uniform approach to the collection of data. This will ensure comparabilty across the district and so allow the exchange of useful data. It might also help to ensure equity of care. The WHO DiabCare Dataset[16] which was developed to monitor the St Vincent Declaration targets is too demanding for current needs and has accordingly been modified by the British Diabetic Association (BDA) and the Audit Group of the Royal College of Physicians of London (RCP)[17] . This modified version*, which has been approved by the Diabetes and Endocrinology Committee of the RCP, has the added advantage that it is simpler and has three levels of entry, but does not conform to the new Read Coding System. Although this modified version is acceptable to diabetologists the relevant committees of the Royal College

* Colloquially known as UK modified DiabCare DataSet

of General Practitioners (RCGP) and the the British Medical Association's GMSC only see a use for entry level one in general practice[18].

Issue for health authority consideration:

a) Which dataset is best?
Currently no single dataset is being used nationally. Only entry level one of the UK modified DiabCare DataSet, advocated by the BDA, has found favour with the RCGP and the GMSC.

5 Confidentiality

Patients have a right to privacy no more so than when they are ill. It is a central tenet of the Patient's Charter that ..."*everyone working in the NHS is under a legal duty to keep your records confidential"*[19] The Data Protection Act of 1984[20] is meant to safeguard all computerised data as does the EC Directive on Data Protection[21], which was adopted in July 1995 and which must be implemented by 1998. Professional colleagues are aware of the need for patient confidentiality and to a greater or lesser extent have arrangements in place to ensure that it is observed at all times. Guidance on the implementation of the Data Protection Act has already been given by the Department of Health[22] who will also be issuing definitive guidance for the NHS on the protection and use of patient information in March 1996.[23]

Patients must be aware that they are on a register and the purpose of the register explained. Information about individual patients held on a register may only be passed on by the health authority, to a third party, on a need to know basis for a specific essential purpose and usually only with the patient's consent.

Issues for health authority consideration:

a) Do patients need to be told that they are on a register.
Yes, and the purpose of the register must be explained.

b) Can patient information be passed on to a third party if it is anonymised?
Yes. However, patients must normally be made aware that this is necessary for a particular purpose. It is important to remember also that a) anonymising information does not of itself remove the duty of confidence; and b) simply removing a patients' name or other identifying data may not do enough to ensure that he or she cannot be traced.
The legal responsibility for the use and ultimate security of the information rests with the health authority.

Conclusion

The NHS Executive agrees in principle that properly constructed and maintained district population-based registers can facilitiate the delivery of targeted, evidence-based, and cost effective specialist care which would be likely i) to improve local arrangements for the provision of care ii) ensure the appropriate levels of provision and iii) enable the delivered care to be reviewed at general practice and at health authority levels. If district population-based registers can achieve these objectives then improvements in clinical outcomes would probably be achieved, if not directly then indirectly, by providing the best possible scenario for the delivery of a good quality service. However, as yet there is no evidence which supports this hypothesis and so justify the additional expenditure. In addition, although some general practices are happy to provide data for district registers on a continuous basis they only represent a small proportion of the whole.

Before making a decison to set up district registers health authorities will have to consider carefully the implications for general practitioners, who will be expected to provide much of the data. There are also important issues of concern to individual members of the public regarding privacy and choice which underpin and extend beyond the statutory issues of data handling. In considering such sensitivities it is important to avoid arousing feelings of health "police". Hence the emphasis which primary care places on the participation of GP practices, where a population focus can occur which is manifestly both user friendly and tailored to the needs of patients and their carers. In attempting to engage and sustain the interest of practices in this approach, it is important to avoid duplication of effort which could result in excessive bureaucracy, which the "Patients not Paper" initiative has sought to reduce. It would be unfortunate if something so important as diabetic care reversed this trend.

To encourage the development of registers in secondary care might also dilute the clear message to general practice that such registers are important and best provided by practices themselves, grouping together and collaborating, when they are confident that they have the resources to do this competently. Thus it could be regarded that the introduction of a second focus for disease management registration within a district at this time might be unhelpful, resulting in a dilution of effort, possible patient antagonism and potentially leading to an increase in GP bureaucracy at a time when other methods have been taken to reduce it.

Thus before making any decision health care planners will have to address the following

> ***Ten Key Questions:–***
> - is a district population-based register necessary?
> - is it likely to improve clinical outcomes?
> - is it a cost effective way of improving clinical outcomes?
> - can confidentiality and security of the data be guaranteed?
> - will the additional data collection place unnecessary burdens on GPs?
> - are patients aware of the register and its purpose?
> - will it assist the strategic planning of the service?
> - is the information technology which is currently available adequate for this purpose?
> - is the dataset simple and agreed by all parties?
> - should it be disease specific or generic?

References

1   Statement of Fees and Allowances (The Red Book). (1990), para 30 et seq, schedules 4 & 5. *The Chronic Disease Management Programme*

2   Krans, HMJ., Porta, M., Keen, H. Diabetes care and research: The St. Vincent's Declaration Action Programme. *C. Ital. Diabetologia.* 1992.

3   *The Department of Health/British Diabetic Association,* Report of the St. Vincent Joint Task Force for Diabetes. (Department of Health/British Diabetic Association, 1995)

4   *Clinical Standards Advisory Group:* "Standards of Clinical Care for people with Diabetes." (HMSO,1994)

5   ibid. Home, P.

6   ibid. Cheales, N. A.

7   ibid. Young, R. J.

8   ibid. Vaughan, N. J. A.

9   North West Regional Health Authority: Personal Communication

10 ibid. Dickinson, F.

11 North West Regional Health Authority: Personal Communication

12 Personal Communication

13 NHS-Wide Networking Programme—NHS Wide Networking Security Project. Security Guide for IM & T specialists. (Department of Health, 1995)

14 General Medical Practice Computer Systems. Requirements for Accreditation Version 3 1995/96 (NHS Excutive 1995)

15 Model Practice on Information Security (NHS Exectuive, 1995)

16 Piwernetz, K., Home, P. D., Snorgaard, O., Antsiferov, M., Staehr-Johansen, K., Krans, M., *for the DIABCARE Monitoring Group of the St Vincent Declaration Steering Committee.* "Monitoring the targets of the St Vincent declaration and the implementation of quality management in diabetes care: the DIABCARE initiative." *Diabetic Medicine* 10 (1993), 371–377

17 Vaughan, N. J. A., Home, P. D., *for the Diabetes Audit Working Group of the Research Unit of the Royal College of Physicians and the British Diabetic Association.* "The UK diabetes dataset." *Diabetic Medicine* 12 (1995), 717–722

18 Royal College of General Practitioners/British Medical Association: Personal Communication

19 Patients Charter and You. (Department of Health, 1995)

20 The Data Protection Act (HMSO, 1984)

21 EC Data Protection Directive, 95/46/EC

22 DH guidance on Data Protection Act, Department of Health: Under cover of HC(87)14; HC(87)26; and HC(89)29.

23 The Protection and Use of Patient Information. Guidance from the Department of Health.(Under cover of HSG(96)18)

1.4 The Economic Issues Regarding Patient Registers

Francis Dickinson, Economic Adviser, Economic and Operational Research Division, Department of Health, London

Introduction

There are four main steps in an economic appraisal of patient registers:–
- definition of the **aims and objectives**;
- setting out the alternative options for achieving these including the present system. The options could be in terms of, for example, the size, scope, location and/or the method of delivery of registers;
- assessing the costs and the benefits of each option over the lifetime of the investment;

and
- considering how costs and benefits will be shared between patients, the NHS, and other organisations.

Aims and Objectives

A possible objective is to have a comprehensive, accurate population-based register in order to:–
- provide appropriate care to all known diabetics (eg regular episodes of care, routine monitoring and follow–up, screening);
- enable all providers involved in shared care to have sufficient information to contact and treat patients;
- be able to measure targets;

and
- have an accurate and complete patient list for research and evaluation of existing and new treatments.

Alternatives

There are a probably a number of alternative register systems, including:
- GP-based registers
- Hospital-based registers
- District-based registers

and
- Regional/National registers

These should, if possible, be compared against an existing (paper-based) system.

Optional Appraisal

This stage is primarily about trying to identify and measure the costs and benefits for all options on a comprehensive basis, and providing a valid comparison of the options.

Benefits

Ultimately we are concerned with health gain, usually measured in terms of Quality Adjusted Life Years (QALYs) or other similar measures. However we are also interested in the distribution of QALYs, eg do a small number of people benefit in a substantial way or is the benefit thinly and widely spread.

Benefits are likely to be in terms of:
- Timely interventions (episodes of care, screening) and the avoidance of complications;
- In the long-run, improved treatments resulting from research;
- Possible spin-off benefits, eg better-informed GPs;
- Reducing duplication between different providers;

and
- Reducing the costs of existing paper-based methods.

Costs

For all alternatives, these are likely to include:–
- Set-up costs (eg for district register, it has been suggested that these are likely to be of the order of £30,000–£50,000, mainly hardware, software, IT support and training);
- On-going costs (eg for district register, this might be one person (Whole Time Equivalent) at say £20,000 annually, including a small allowance for on-costs);
- Other register costs (eg future upgrading, enhancements, networking, etc):
- Private costs, in particular costs incurred by GPs, carers and patients (eg time, transport).

One needs to be mindful of possible hidden costs, and for example cost escalation normally associated with computerised systems. On the other hand, the potential benefits of computerisation are also difficult to anticipate comprehensively. This uncertainty is best dealt with using sensitivity analysis, which involves varying key assumptions to see whether this has any impact on the ranking of options.

Timing of Costs and Benefits

Costs and benefits need to be measured and evaluated over the lifetime of investments, not just the immediate costs and benefits. The time profile of costs and benefits might also be important since it may be differ between options, especially if options vary in terms of level of technology or the trade-off between initial investment and maintenance. Where an investment has a significant lifetime, it is necessary to apply a discount factor to reflect the fact that more distant (ie later) costs and benefits are of lower present value than those occurring immediately.

Risks

Often, more ambitious projects based on newer technology are more risky, in the sense that there is a higher probability that benefits will turn out lower than expected and/or costs higher than expected. It is therefore useful to identify those factors which have most influence on costs and benefits and assess how much these would need to change to alter the choice of preferred option (ie risk analysis).

Issues

Likely Size

An important factor is the projected size of register(s). For diabetes, given that the prevalence is say up to 2% of the population, the total number registered in England at any one time is likely to be about 1,000,000 patients.

On a district basis, there are currently about 93 districts with populations ranging between about 200,000 and 1,000,000. This suggests that district registers would probably range in size between about 4,000 and 20,000 patients per register.

Other relevant factors will be:–
- the extent of movement of patients between registers;
- which organisations/providers need access to the register, and how might this best be managed.

Other issues impacting on the economic justification for registers include:
- Sources of information for establishing Registers;
- NHS information management issues, such as the impact of the new patient number;
- incentives/disincentives to establish/maintain Registers;
- level of expertise and training required;
- last but not least, the arrangements in each area between provider units, DHAs, and GPs.

1.5   Data Currently Available to the Department of Health on Diabetes

David Hewitt, Statistician, Department of Health, London

Introduction

This paper reviews data currently collected by the Department, with particular reference to diabetes. My role in the Department is that of Statistician responsible for statistics on hospital activity and facilities. These include data from the Hospital Episode Statistics system but other sources will also be discussed.

Hospital Episode Statistics (HES)

Hospital Episode Statistics, or HES, is the successor to the Hospital In-patient Enquiry, or HIPE, which was discontinued in 1985. HES started life in 1987 as a consequence of the recommendations of the Korner Committee which reviewed NHS information in the 1980s. HES is a by-product of hospital systems for administering patients, and is built up from individual records as patients progress through hospital.

Until this year, information from patient records was sent to the Office of Population Censuses and Surveys, OPCS. Individual records were anonymised to protect patient confidentiality, and a random 1–in–4 sample was taken which became the basis of the published HES data. Volumes have been published for each year from 1988–89 to 1993–94. For each year, the raw figures have been adjusted, first, because not all episodes were covered, and secondly because, of those episodes that were covered, not all had a valid diagnosis.

Coverage in terms both of overall episodes and of diagnosis has improved greatly over the first 6 years of HES: in 1988–89 overall coverage was 95%, of which only 74% had a valid diagnosis; by 1993–94 overall coverage had gone up to 99.6%, of which 96% had a valid diagnosis.

The basic unit by which we measure hospital activity is the Consultant Episode. This is defined as the period of time spent under the care of one lead consultant in one health care provider. This was the unit adopted by the Korner Committee as being best able to provide an accurate measure of consultant workload.

In 1993, HES was market tested. The 5–year contract was won by the Company Data Sciences, who are now responsible for processing HES data for 1994–95 and subsequent years. The new system has been designed to be more user-friendly than the earlier one, with Department staff having access to screens on which they can browse through HES data. Users can also design statistical tables using a "mini" data-base. When users have decided exactly what they want a table to look like, they can send instructions for the Company's mini-computer to access the full data set of around 10 million episodes a year, produce the required table, and then send it back down the line.

As regards diabetes and its complications, HES data shows that between 1989–90 and 1993–94 the number of episodes of diabetes mellitus went up from 52 to 58 thousand. Within the total, there was a fall in the number of episodes without any complications (these fell from 28 to 19 thousand). There was a particular increase in the number of cases with ophthalmic complications, which went up from 8 to 15 thousand.

We can also link episodes with a particular operation to those with a specific diagnosis, and hence look at amputation operations where the main diagnosis was diabetes mellitus. These increased by about 50% between 1989–90 and 1993–94, from an estimated 1,335 to 1,930. The limbs most frequently affected were the leg (926 in 1993–94) and the toe (812). As these figures are based on the 1 in 4 sample, they must all be regarded as having a margin of error. Our knowledge will improve when (for 1994–95) HES moves on to a 100% basis.

As data quality continues to improve, we will be able to analyse data for smaller areas, such as DHA areas and also produce data at provider level. The Department is currently developing protocols to ensure that confidentiality is maintained, and it is envisaged that data will not be released when it represents fewer than 10 episodes. Highly sensitive areas, such as AIDS and STDs, will continue to receive the greatest protection, and data for these topics will be aggregated to a much higher level.

Uses of HES Data

The tables and chart below, which are based on data from HES, show recent trends in hospital admissions for diabetes and its complications and in related operative procedures.

FINISHED CONSULTANT EPISODES (Ordinary admissions plus day cases)
ENGLAND, 1989-90 to 1993-94
(Source: Department of Health, Hospital Episode Statistics)

DIABETES MELLITUS AND COMPLICATIONS
('000)

ICD9 codes	Complications	1989-90	1993-94
250.0	None	28.4	19.5
250.1	Ketoacidosis	5.7	6.6
250.2	Coma	1.1	1.1
250.3	Renal	1.2	1.5
250.4	Ophthalmic	8.2	15.4
250.5	Neurological	1.1	1.1
250.6	Peripheral circulatory disorders	3.9	5.1
250.7	Other specified	0.4	1.5
250.9	Unspecified	1.9	6.6
	Total	51.9	58.4

DIABETES MELLITUS ADMISSIONS - COMPLICATIONS

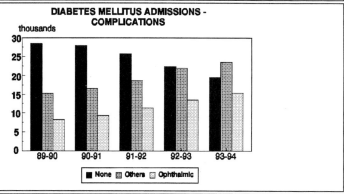

■ None ▨ Others ▨ Ophthalmic

NUMBER OF AMPUTATION OPERATIONS WITH MAIN DIAGNOSIS OF DIABETES MELLITUS

Operation codes	Affected limb	1989-90	1990-91	1991-92	1992-93	1993-94
X07	Arm	0	0	0	4	4
X08	Hand	8	4	4	8	4
X09	Leg	603	776	844	915	926
X10	Foot	108	135	160	171	155
X11	Toe	578	571	760	757	812
X12	Amputation stump	37	13	17	29	29
	Total	1,335	1,500	1,785	1,884	1,930

Data from General Practitioners

There are two sources of data from general practitioners (GPs), the Royal College of General Practitioners (RCGP) weekly returns and the national study of Morbidity Statistics from General Practice, or MSGP, which takes place every 10 years. The latest one, known as MSGP4, relates to 1991–92.

The RCGP surveys obtain weekly figures from a panel of GPs across the country. The RCGP currently collects data under 26 headings for communicable diseases and 18 headings (including diabetes) for non-communicable diseases.

MSGP4 covers 1% of the population and provides information on consulting rates, prevalence and first incidence at each level of diagnostic detail, which are in many cases linked with patients' socio-economic data. The summary report for the chapter on **Endocrine, nutritional and metabolic diseases** comments:

> "Diabetes was the most common condition in this chapter. One per cent of the sample consulted for this. Although the rate of newly-diagnosed cases of diabetes declined since 1981–82, the proportion of people with diabetes increased over this period. A high proportion consulted for obesity, acquired hypothyroidism and gout."

The Health Survey for England

The Health Surveys for England do not reach people via hospital episodes or GP consultations, but by a direct survey of individuals. The main aim of the Health Surveys of 1991 to 1993 has been to obtain information on aspects of health relevant to cardiovascular disease (CVD). The major risk factors for CVD have been identified as smoking, hypertension, raised plasma cholesterol and inadequate physical activity. Diabetes is a contributory factor, along with obesity, excessive alcohol consumption, and high salt intake.

In the 1991 Survey respondents (who were aged 16 and over) were asked whether they had ever been diagnosed as diabetic. Among men with 3 or 4 of the major risk factors for CVD, 5% had diabetes. Of those with fewer than 3 risk factors only 1% were diabetic. The pattern among women was similar.

In 1992 and 1993 the investigation of diabetes was extended by testing sampled blood for blood glucose [a level of over 5.2% being diagnostic of diabetes]. The results suggested that between 3 and 4 per cent of the population are at risk of developing diabetes—particularly those who are older and obese. These people often have other risk factors for CVD such as raised blood pressure or physical inactivity.

Fourth National Survey of Ethnic Minorities

The Fourth National Survey is the latest in a series carried out by the Policy Studies Institute on ethnic minorities in England and Wales, and is the first to contain questions on health. The sample comprises 5,000 members of ethnic minorities and a comparison sample of 2,500 whites.

The Fourth Survey included 2 items specifically about diabetes. One asked whether respondents had any of five specified conditions, of which one was diabetes. The other was a follow-up to affirmative answers, asking whether the respondent attended a diabetes clinic. There was also a question about medicines. The findings of the Survey are due to be published next summer, and will throw light on the prevalence of diabetes in a number of ethnic minority groups and in whites, and on their use of diabetes treatment clinics and of medication.

1.6   Confidentiality* and Medical Registers

Professor Roger Higgs, King's College School of Medicine and Dentistry, Department of General Practice and Primary Care, King's College, London

Introduction

IAGO: Good name in man and woman dear my lord,
Is the immediate jewel of their souls.
Who steals my purse, steals trash; 'tis something, nothing;
'Twas mine, 'tis his, and has been slave to thousands:
But he that filches from me my good name
Robs me of that which not enriches him
And makes me poor indeed.   *(Shakespeare: Othello)*

What happens when people learn things about us which we should rather they did not know?

The problem of maintaining confidentiality in the face of increased sharing of information through electronic links is not confined to medicine, but has an urgency in health care now because of particular circumstances and needs. The arguments pull both ways. On the one hand, it is now understood that collected data is vital in all aspects of medicine, in personal care as well as public health, as a source of responses based on evidence and for the most effective deployment of the resources available. On the other, confidentiality in the transactions between an individual and a professional is so basic to health care, that it could almost be seen as a marker of the work itself. The ability of a patient to speak openly, without fear of information being passed on, is common to all healing work worldwide and throughout the ages, and is as much part of the fabric of medical work as the finger on the pulse or the hand on the belly. We no longer swear the Hippocratic Oath, but the sense of it continues to underpin medicine. "All that comes to my knowledge in the exercise of my profession, or outside of my profession, or in my daily commerce with people, which ought not to be spread abroad, I will keep secret and never reveal." The statement is clear.

Yet even before the ink is dry or the stethescope is laid on the desk, we know that this promise is problematical. Difficulties arise well before registers or electronic connections are considered. Public policy, for instance, may require a different approach, as in child abuse. The requirement to

* The Department of Health will be issuing new guidance on confidentiality in March 1996

break medical confidence may even be expressed in law, as in dealing with an injured terrorist. The complexities of modern health care may appear to make confidentiality impossible: in a well known article, Siegler described how over 100 people had legitimate access to the patient's chart in hospital[1]. Add to that the leakiness of any system, and claims of public interest (often masking people's deep love of scandal), and the sun appears to set on the Hippocratic tradition. It could be seen, as Siegler suggested, as a "decrepit concept".

So before we can make progress, we have to examine and resolve some of these problems. We need to bring together the tradition and its modern applications, the theory and current practice. We should examine where the concept comes from, possible exceptions to it, and how we should handle them, before coming to the specific issue of registers.

Privacy

Lying behind all our ideas about confidentiality, lies the suggestion that human beings do, in some sense, have a right to maintain some things as private in any humane society. The exclusion of others from one's personal area can work both ways. In reminding Othello of this, Iago was also cleverly suggesting that he knew something powerful and sinister about which he would rather not speak; from playground days onwards, we know that a whispered secret immediately creates outside interest. But privacy as a concept suggests something more—that there is an area in human life which is not only nobody else's business, but which actually *requires* to be kept secret for human life to work at all. For instance, in spite of our more relaxed approach these days, it is still the case that few of us would be able to have rewarding sexual relationships or develop intimate partnerships without privacy. It has been suggested in the western world, that this right should be protected by law (especially in view of the recent increased intrusion of the media into the private lives of public figures). In an article discussing privacy, the American lawyer, Charles Fried, developed this in the medical field.

> We may not mind that a person knows a general fact about us, yet feel our privacy invaded if he knows the details. For instance, a casual acquaintance may comfortably know that I am sick, but it could violate my privacy if he knows the nature of that illness. Or a good friend may know what particular illness I am suffering from, but it would violate my privacy if he were actually to witness my suffering from some symptom which he must know is associated with the disease[2].

Thus whether there is or is not such a right of privacy, we all certainly have a feeling of needing to preserve some of our lives from instrusion. Confidentiality then develops from those areas we choose to keep in the private sphere and depends on an understanding that this privacy is vital for human life as we know it. These concepts become critical just because doctors and other health care workers have, in order to do their work, to probe into bodies, ask about personal behaviour and attitudes, discuss experiences and so on: to enter precisely these areas which we should normally wish to be maintained (and in healthy society, many would consider, should be maintained) in the private sphere. The medical "secret" is thus intrinsic to the work; and that it remain a shared secret, requires confidentiality.

An Unbreakable Rule?

Many commentators have suggested that there should be no exceptions to this principle, and that a medical secret once imparted, should be maintained completely and forever. This is certainly backed by French law[3] and has received strong support from the venereal disease legislation in this country and in the handling of the AIDS epidemic. The case is put well by Professor Anthony Pinching in his piece "AIDS: Health Care Ethics & Society"[4]. But others would maintain that there have to be exceptions to an absolute interpretation: this is accepted by the General Medical Council, and sometimes, as we have seen, appears to be required by law.

But there are more everyday examples. Modern health care is not delivered by individuals but by teams. Information has to be shared. Professionals working with families, especially in primary care, face similar problems. Boundaries may be loose and changing, and confidential work here requires sensitive judgement. In a multicultural and plurilingual society, interpreters of all sorts are needed and these often come from within the family. Thus the professional/family boundary is blurred. At a recent conference in New Zealand, a South Sea Island health care worker made a dramatic appeal to doctors to understand this need and stop excluding her from discussions with relatives; in her case, she felt she was the interpreter, both culturally and linguistically, to no less than 120 people in her extended family. Placing the cordon of secrecy outside such a professional group, and including the other workers involved, is a possible answer, in practice. But whatever is decided, a policy and practice is required which is sensitive to particular situations and individual needs. How can this be done without sacrificing the central rule?

Four Principles

One way is to use the now well known approach through four principles which has been developed in USA and UK in the work of Beauchamp and Chidress[5] and Gillon. This suggests that conflicts can be clarified by looking at the important principles behind them, and has outlined four of especial importance: **respect for autonomy, doing good or beneficence, avoiding or minimising harm (non-maleficence), and justice**. Confidentiality is derived from the need to respect a person's choice as to what should be shared from his or her personal and medical secrets. Just as consent would normally be required for a doctor to intrude physically (otherwise a medical touching risks becoming an assault), so consent is needed for the passing on of information which arises from such contact. The principle of beneficence would back this up—normally such behaviour would benefit the patient. But not always; a psychotic crisis might be a counter-example, and under the principle of non-maleficence, we have seen that in child abuse cases, workers may have to break confidence if major harm is to be prevented. In psychological work, the classic case was that of Tatiana Tarasoff, a Californian student whose life was at risk from a man in therapy; in this context, the man suggested he really wanted to kill Tatiana. Because this information was not responded to (although attempts were made), he succeeded in carrying out his threat. In the subsequent case brought by Tatiana's parents against the University, the Judge declared against the claim for preserving professional confidentiality that "the protective privilege ends where the public peril begins"[6]. Here confidentiality was seen as a privilege to be waived in some serious circumstances, not a right to be maintained at all times. The principle of justice here required that the application of a medical rule be fair to all those involved: and breaking professional confidence was considered a minor harm when set against the threat of murder.

Perspectives and Values

Further work in which I am involved suggests that the application and sorting of these principles usually involves us in more detailed, and often extremely complex choices; we take into consideration the views of all those involved in a transaction, for instance, and the values of the particular system in which we are operating. In the first case, we would need to see how different stakeholders viewed the balance of principles in a particular decision. As to values, even different parts of the same may have different priorities. Thus, general practice may respond positively to the needs of a family, public health may wish to examine the evidence that such an action may be cost-effective, a hospital specialist may be required, first and foremost, to exclude serious illness, and so on. Each person, and each branch of medical work, will, of necessity, need to make a slightly different balance of judgements, depending on the task with which it is entrusted. This is not to say that the principles are constantly flexible, but that their interpretation and enactment is initially dependant on the context. This gives policymakers and, in particular, policymakers for inter-connecting groups or systems, particular problems. This suggests that confidentiality, if it is not an absolute principle, has to be handled with sensitivity and judgement in the context of the personal care of that particular patient.

The Problem for Registers

Immediately this raises a series of issues for those planning registers. Can the information be anonymous or unattributable? If not, the following must be considered:–

1 The register may take information *completely out of context*, and may land it, if attributed, in a situation where, at best, good judgements cannot be made about its sensitivity and importance, and, at worst, where it may be abused. The individual can no longer negotiate how, and to whom, this information is passed. He is, as it were, naked in public; it is a nightmare we all dread. The smallest disability may be of completely different significance out of context. The normal negotiation of consent becomes impossible.

2 *The information may be wrong.* Creating registers is one thing, maintaining them is another. A person may have a loss of consciousness which evidence indicates is due to epilepsy. Later evidence may emerge that it was due to another cause, but how is the label changed? Some labels are very "sticky" because of the emotional value attached to them in society, yet we know that diagnoses, and even some laboratory tests, are facts based on probability. Even some cancers may be incorrectly diagnosed. If facts are wrong, how is this corrected?

3 Registers are notoriously *difficult to change*, partly due to the above, but partly because they may take on an objective life of their own, and people rightly have the greatest reluctance in tampering with them or changing information contained in them. Most computer systems have a trace in them which means that information once put in, can, baring accidents, always be retrieved. Human life goes through stages and attitudes change; we are not concerned, perhaps, that a particular politician wet the bed when a very young child, but we might be that he or she had used cannabis. Yet for the average South London adolescent, depending on age, the second would, currently, be so common as to be normal, while the first might be a sign of gross psychological disturbance. As the person grows up and conquers these habits, how is a register changed?

4 Registers may be *hard to police*, especially if held electronically. My news this week tells me that the Government in UK, no less, has a project in hand which will, if successful, enable it to hack into all available electronic systems. Organisations have long known that lists, addresses and so on are prone to burglary, and take precautions. But burglary, at least, once it happens is usually known, and people can be informed that personal information is "out". Electronic hacking of some types may not be detectable.

5 It is usually the *responsibility* of the person or organisation to whom information is given to maintain the safety of that information. (We should not blame someone who took reasonable precautions, but whose office was burgled). But if as a routine, or part of a network, this information is passed, the responsibility begins to blur.

Practical Suggestions

Thus, a second set of practical suggestions begins to emerge when we try to set the issues of medical confidentiality in the context of registers. Rather than an absolute principle, we see the judgement to be one about *stringency*. How strict must we be in which context? This must be considered for all angles, and by all involved in the use of registers, but in particular the question of consent of those whose information is on the system requires a lot of work and cannot be taken for granted. New methods need to be developed here.

Secondly, *safeguards* are vital and need to be constantly examined. Once a system becomes untrustworthy, it becomes useless. But the risks are both general and personal. Everyone has his or her own risk list or set of priorities. A comedian may make huge use in her professional life of her own personal material; a psychiatrist probably would not. Equally, if there is a mistake, someone must be able to be *responsible* and held *accountable*; and redress, if required, must be obtainable. Linked to this, therefore, is a new campaign of *personal and public awareness*. The person who puts information into a register must know exactly what it is to be used for, where it will go, but so must the person whose information is being added. This proposes a considerable barrier to effective or efficient health care, whichever way it is examined. Currently, it would be safe to assume that very little is said to a health care user about placing data on a register. But to change this may change the pattern of health care; as a doctor, if I take even five minutes explaining the system to my patient, that five minutes is lost to other forms of health care work I might have done instead.

Thus since the inclusion of a particular patient on a register requires consent from that patient, and consent requires explanation, the cost benefit equation is not between "discussion and a no discussion" but between "register and no register", or a variant of this. The opportunity costs are vital to assess. For instance, do the benefits of the register justify this cost in terms of use of a professional's time? Also, if we are to take evidence-based medicine as seriously as is required, it will be necessary to *demonstrate the real benefits of registers*. It will not be enough to be enthusiastic about registers, without also being able to show how they help public health and personal health care, and in this equation, what are the gains and losses in each sphere. Ultimately, there may be some judgement and choices to be made, which might lead to the conclusion that too much may be lost by certain types of information sharing. Just as the best surgeon may reluctantly decide to spare the knife, so the best health service planner or manager may withhold the register.

Such apparently negative talk does not derive from a direct assessment of confidentiality problems however, so much as from an academic's requirement to test and justify new routines. Confidentiality remains an issue for registers, but, in my view, a soluble one, provided that appropriate complexity of information is included, personal relationships are respected and anonymity is assured, unless proper consent is given. There are regulations and there may be laws which bear on this, which should be explored more deeply than I am able to. But registers are a means to good health care, not an end in themselves; the register is for man, and not man for the register. In this regard *confidentiality should be considered as a powerful tradition, hard to keep in good order but only to be broken by agreement for overriding reasons on good evidence.*

References

1   Siegler, M., "Confidentiality in medicine: a decrepit concept." *New England Journal of Medicine* 307 (1982), 1518–21

2   Fried, C., "Privacy: a Rational Context." *Yale Law Journal* 77 (1968) 475–93

3   Gillon, R., *Philosophical Medical Ethics.* (Wiley Chichester, 1985), 106

4   Chapter in Gillon, R., *Principles of Health Care Ethics.* (Wiley Chichester, 1994)

5   Beauchamp, T., Childress, J., *Principles of Biomedical Ethics.* (Oxford University Press New York, 1989)

6   op. cit. Beauchamp, T., Childress, J., 402

1.7 Diabetes Registers: The Nursing Contribution

Simon Old, Nursing Officer, NHS Executive, Leeds

Introduction

The use of registers in a multiprofessional primary health care environment will be maximised if there is recognition of the valuable contributions that can be made by each member of the primary health care team. Nurses and health visitors in all settings can make an important contribution to the collection and use of the data required to support diabetes registers. Practice nurses, district nurses, health visitors, hospital nurses on the wards or in clinics and the growing number of specialist nurses all have their part to play if patients are to receive the most appropriate care through the use of diabetes registers.

The majority of people, together with their family or friends, have to manage their own care and treatment for most of the time. In the task force report on nursing in primary health care "New World, new opportunities"[1] the task group returned again and again to the importance of teamwork. Teamwork, with shared vision, shared objectives and where appropriate shared protocols was seen as essential if the range of skills, and the resources to deploy them, were to be channelled to the maximum benefit. This is particularly relevant when considering the needs of people with long term conditions such as diabetes. Primary health care nursing is distinguished by its emphasis on guiding and supporting clients in their care, involving them as partners at every stage. It also involves promoting healthy lifestyles and ensuring that services are targeted to those needing them most.

Data Collection and Use

Data quality is vital in securing the benefits from the use of a register. One important premise in assuring data quality is to ensure that data collectors are data users. They at the very least need to understand and value the benefits derived from using the data they are collecting. It is also important for the client and data collector to have a good rapport and a mutual understanding of the value of the register. Thus it is likely that every member of the primary health care team will find themselves in the appropriate circumstances to be both data collectors and users.

When considering the role of nurses in the data collection process several factors need to be considered. In the context of diabetes, information needs are well understood. The St Vincent Declaration[2] embodies a commitment to continuous quality improvement and the implementation of the targets embodied in it requires the systematic monitoring of the key quality indicators of diabetes care. To achieve thorough monitoring there is both the need for diabetes registers based on agreed national datasets and the use of information technology.

The recommended data set associated with the St Vincent Declaration is appropriate for personal diabetes status records for patients, quality assurance by health care providers, service planning by health care providers and commissioners, contract monitoring and national aggregation for monitoring and external comparison. This variety of uses is both important to the data sets perceived value by those collecting the data and also in considering how best it may be captured and used. One of the major problems highlighted by community providers is the requirement for nurses and health visitors to collect specific data for a single purpose when that same data has little or no use for the operational staff. Fortunately the breadth of the St Vincent approach ensures that this is not the case in respect of their proposed diabetes minimum data set. However when planning the local approach to data collection the community Information Systems for Providers project[3] identified some clear principles which are worthy of note:
- information needed for management purposes should be produced as a byproduct of operational systems,
- data should help staff to monitor input and clinical outcomes and to examine and improve clinical effectiveness, and
- the workload imposed by data collection and analysis should not detract from patient care.

If nurses are appropriately empowered to deliver education and direct care they will play a vital role in collecting accurate data. It must be recognised that a register is a means not an end and that the nursing contribution is not confined to data collection. Sheffield Health Authority[4] advocated the setting up and monitoring of a district diabetes protocol. Services should be district wide, integrated and specialist led. Collaboration will thus be the key element at all levels and the patient's needs fundamental to the philosophy of care.

As a primary care led NHS becomes a reality and with more care being delivered in the community we have to enable the generalist. There is a fine balance between the role of specialists and generalists in care. The diabetes specialist nurse/health visitor working as part of an outreach service as an extension of hospital secondary care can play an important role in bridging the specialist, generalist gap. Powerful communication protocols are also an important tool to enable generalists

Lawrence[5] suggests that the increasing numbers of practice nurses yields a unique opportunity to expand in-practice care and specialist nurse facilitators could lend appropriate expertise support and audit direction. Nurses as lead clinicians is not a new concept and nurse/health visitor led clinics can make a significant contribution to the delivery of care and client education.

Information Technology

There are significant advantages of registers being computerised and available to nurses and other users. A computerised diabetic register could support recall requirements, screening, and health education by linking guidelines and protocols to the register.

Information systems are required in the operational environment to support:
- the operational care of the patient,
- contracting and resource management and
- the production of comparative management information

In addition there are four areas where information will be of prime importance:
- local use of information, to strengthen local management including clinical audit and indicators of quality,
- NHS wide use of information for exchange and comparison,
- contracting and the flow of data from providers to commissioners to accompany contracts and
- central uses of information to enable national trends to be assessed and monitored and to enable future policy development.

Wherever possible data should only be collected once and then through the appropriate and safe use of technology shared as required. Thus in information technology terms it may neither be necessary or desirable to develop discrete diabetic register systems. In circumstances where person based clinical systems are already in use the diabetic register data set could be a natural bi-product of the operational system which could support screening, recall and provide protocol support to operational procedures and patient education.

Appropriate technology and a consistent, shared minimum data set could offer:
- improved efficiency of data collection when data is collected only once
- improved quality of service delivery for the patient who only has to give information once
- better identification of individual patients so that health events and episodes of care may be linked.

The IM&T Strategy[6] launched in 1992 proposed that the service should work towards having secure, integrated, person based, operational Information technology. Nationally this has been facilitated by the development of common clinical terms, the unique person identifier or NHS number, national data and communications standards, the NHS Administrative Register and the NHS-wide network.

Although advocating a person centred approach to data collection it is important that minimum data sets allow flexibility in approaches to service delivery. In particular we must guard against specified data sets erecting artificial barriers around particular services or individuals. For example it is important not to have barriers around professional groups who are providing a collaborative service package to an individual, or between hospital based care and domiciliary based care.

Many in community will not currently have the required technology to meet their needs. In such cases simple registration and collection forms are essential. There is scope in hospital clinics an general practices to modify current registers and produce basic new databases to allow retrieval. However if the full benefits of registers are to be achieved the future must be towards information systems providing decision support and protocol led advice. If nurses and health visitors are to make the fullest possible contribution to patient care then they need to be enabled by having available appropriate technology at the point of care delivery.

References

1 "New world, new opportunities: Nursing in primary health care" (NHS Executive, 1993)

2 *World Health Organisation (Europe) and International Diabetes Federation (Europe).* "Diabetes care and research in Europe: the St Vincent declaration." *Diabetic Medicine* 7 (1990), 360

3 Community Information Systems for Providers, Describing Community Care. Final Report. (NHS Executive, 1993)

4 "People with diabetes mellitus: a strategy for health services." (Sheffield Health Authority, 1993)

5 Lawrence, J. R., "Shared diabetic care." *British Journal of Hospital Medicine* vol 48, no 1 (1992), 34–39

6 An Information Management and Technology Strategy for the NHS in England. "Getting better with information." (NHS Executive, 1992)

1.8 Diabetes Registers—A Personal View of a Purchaser

Dr Margaret Guy, Consultant in Public Health Medicine, Brent and
Harrow Health Authority, Harrow, Midddlesex

Introduction

This presentation focuses on diabetes registers from the perspective of a Consultant in Public Health Medicine working within a health authority.

The role of the New Health Authorities

As from April 1996 District Health Authorities (DHAs) and Family Health Services Authorities (FHSAs) will be replaced by new unitary Health Authorities which will be responsible for implementing national health policy at a local level. Their overall aim will be to maximise the health of the local population within available resources.

The anticipated role of these new health authorities has been set out in the NHS Executive circular EL(94)79. Health authorities will be responsible for:–

- Monitoring the health of the local population and assessing their health care needs
- Identifying local health priorities in consultation with the local community
- Developing local strategies and policies to address these identified priorities in partnership with GP Fundholders, local providers of health care and other local organisations whose actions impact on the health of the local population, including local authorities and voluntary organisations.
- Overseeing the implementation of these strategies and policies—this will include ensuring that there is an equitable distribution of available resources and equal access to health care services
- Monitoring the impact of these strategies and policies on the health of the population.

Developing Local Diabetes Strategies

In order to develop and implement strategies for maximising the health of local residents with diabetes, health authorities will need to be able to:–
- Monitor the health of their diabetic population
- Monitor whether all patients have access to high quality diabetes care
- Monitor the effectiveness of the diabetes care provided.

Information Needs of the Health Authority

Health authorities will therefore need information on:–

- The number of people with diabetes and their demographic characteristics;
  This will enable the prevalence of diabetes in the population as a whole and in subgroups of the population to be monitored;
- The health status of the local diabetic population;
  Ideally health authorities will need to have access to comparable data from other Health Authorities;
- The type and location of health care provided;
  This will enable health authorities to map the current provision of diabetes services;
- The quality of the care provided both in terms of the process and outcomes of the care provided.

Uses of Population-Based Information on People with Diabetes

Access to such information will:–

- Inform the development of local health strategies and health policies;
- Inform the commissioning and development of local services;
- Enable health authorities to set quantified health improvement targets by providing baseline information on the current health status of the diabetic population;
- Enable health authorities to monitor progress towards these agreed targets;
- Enable health authorities to monitor the quality of services provided;
- Allow health authorities to monitor coverage of surveillance programmes, such as diabetic eye screening programmes.

Sources of Information

Health authorities have access to a number of sources of information on the health of the diabetic population and the services provided to them, including:–

1 General Practice

- Data submitted by GPs under the arrangements for the provision of Chronic Disease Management Programmes;
- Data on prescribing by GPs.

2 NHS Trusts

- Data on inpatient admissions;
  Accurate data are available on the number of admissions where diabetes is the main cause of admission, although coding for admissions where

diabetes is a contributory cause of admission is often incomplete.

- Information on the provision of outpatient services;
  It is generally more difficult to obtain data on outpatient care although an increasing number of NHS Trusts are developing hospital-based diabetes registers which can provide very useful information. Provider-based diabetes registers will be discussed in more detail later.
- Information on the provision of community health services;
  Increasingly it is also becoming possible to obtain useful information on services, such as dietetics, chiropody and district nursing services.

3   Optometry Services

FHSAs have information on the number of people with diabetes receiving free eye checks to which they are entitled to annually under the NHS.

4   Local Authority Blindness Registers

Data held on these registers are often incomplete as many people with visual impairment do not wish to be registered and many registers do not include the cause of visual impairment.

5   European Dialysis and Transplant Register

Data are available on the number of people with diabetes who are receiving dialysis and who have undergone a renal transplant.

6   Mortality statistics

Data are available on the number of people who have died as a result of diabetes although, as with data on hospital admissions, recording of diabetes as a contributory cause of death is often incomplete.

Collating Population-Based Information on People with Diabetes

Mechanisms therefore need to be developed to enable Health Authorities to collate information from all of these potential data sources. As a minimum, health authorities will need anonymised data on:–
- the characteristics of people with diabetes;
- the location of their care;
- health outcomes.

NHS providers—GPs and NHS Trusts—will potentially be the main source of the information required to set up population-based diabetes information systems. In effect, health authorities require a subset of the information held on each provider-based register.

Provider-Held Diabetes Registers

Each health service provider needs to have a diabetes register to:–
- Assist the management of individual patients;
- Ensure all patients under the provider's care are receiving regular follow up;
- Assist the planning of service provision, such the frequency and type of clinics provided;
- Facilitate the audit of the quality of care provided, in terms of the process and outcomes of care.

In order to facilitate the collation of useful information at Health Authority level, it will be important to ensure that each provider is collecting comparable data. All providers should therefore be encouraged to use the recommended data set developed by the Working Group set up by the British Diabetic Association (BDA) and the Royal College of Physicians (RCP). This data set includes all the data items required at health authority level. Because of the complexity of the data involved, both the registers held by individual providers and the information collated by health authorities will need to be computerised.

Issues to be addressed when setting up Population-Based Diabetes Information Systems

A number of issues need to be addressed when setting up population-based information systems, including:–

1 Patient Confidentiality

Before people with diabetes are added to any register, they need to be informed that this is happening and be given the option to opt out of being included on the register. It is also important to share the information held on the register with each patient—this can be achieved by recording the information held on the register in a patient-held record card.

Patients need to be reassured that everything is being done to reduce the likelihood of data held on the register being stolen either physically or electronically. Both the security of the building where the computer is housed and the security of computer system itself need to be maximised.

It should be noted that patient confidentiality is not an issue at health authority level if only anonymised data are held. (nb The Department of Health will issue guidance to health authorities on confidentiality issues in March 1996)

2   Ownership of Data held on Registers

Ultimately the data on any register belongs to the patients about whom the data have been collected. At a provider level, the lead health professional involved in the care of the patient should act as the custodian of this information. The Director of Public Health is best placed to act as the custodian of clinical data held on individual patients at a health authority level—Directors of Public Health already act as the custodians of clinical data held on women as part of the Cervical Screening Call/Recall System.

Health professionals are also concerned about the confidentiality of data held on the quality of care they are providing and the potential uses of such information. These concerns can be minimised by promoting the shared ownership of the data by all the health professionals involved.

3   The Initial Setting up of District-based Diabetes Information Systems

Mechanisms need to be put in place to enable the collation at Health Authority level of comparable data from all providers. It will therefore be important to ensure that all providers use the same data set and the same definitions for each data field. As suggested earlier, this can best be achieved if all providers are encouraged to use the BDA/RCP Recommended Data Set.

Each provider will need assistance in identifying all people with diabetes under their care. Even if the necessary resources are identified, we still need to acknowledge that the level of case ascertainment will vary—not all people with diabetes are diagnosed and not all people with diagnosed diabetes are identified. This is a particular issue for patients with diabetes who are not registered with a general practitioner (GP).

When collating general practice data, health authorities will also need to liaise with neighbouring health authorities as some GPs have patients registered on their lists from more than one health authority. In relation to the Chronic Disease Management Programme, GPs currently report on all their patients to the designated Responsible FHSA—inevitably this information will include data on patients from neighbouring FHSAs who may in turn be receiving data on patients outside their area.

When collating data held on hospital-based diabetes registers, health authorities will also need mechanisms to enable them to receive data from all of the providers currently providing care to their residents—providers therefore need to be able to generate district-specific data.

The resources involved in initially setting up provider-based and population-based registers should not be underestimated. Every effort should be made to link in with other data sources.

4 Updating Registers

Having set up a register, it is essential to have mechanisms for updating the register, both in terms of:–

a) The denominator

- Changes in name and/or address;
- Newly diagnosed patients;
- Movements in to and out of the district;
- Deaths.

Systems need to be in place to ensure that newly diagnosed patients are added to registers based in providers and health authorities. Registers which link to the FHSA database will be automatically updated for movements out of the district and for deaths. Where practice databases are electronically linked to the FHSA database, for example as part of the GP Links Project, changes in name and/or address are automatically transferred to the FHSA database and, in turn, can be transferred to the diabetes register. If patients move from another FHSA using the same diabetes information system, data can be automatically added to the receiving Health Authority's information system.

b) Data held on individual patients

Information about patients held on provider-based registers should be updated at least once a year and the Annual Review provides an ideal mechanism for achieving this.

Data held on provider-based registers can either be transferred to health authority based systems by paper or, ideally, electronically. Most systems currently in operation rely on paper transfer of information. This increases the burden for providers of diabetes care in terms of the amount of paper work involved and the costs to health authorities in terms of data entry. A number of initiatives are currently underway which will enable the electronic transfer of data, such as MIQEST, which will enable the downloading of information from GP systems. Again, the task of downloading information will be made easier if all providers use the same data set.

5 Ensuring Data Quality

The quality of the data collected is likely to be higher if it is seen to be useful to the providers of diabetes care. It will therefore be important to ensure that information is fed back to health professionals, for example, as part of an ongoing programme of clinical audit. Sharing of data between health professionals also tends to improve the data quality. The linking of data to resource allocation can also result in improved data completeness although the quality may suffer—financial incentives should only be used as a last resort.

6   Analysis of Data

It will be essential to ensure that aggregated data can be analysed in a useful and meaningful way.

7   Costs of Setting up Running Diabetes Registers

The cost of setting up and running diabetes registers and diabetes information systems will inevitably need to be taken into consideration when advocating the setting up of such systems. The most costly element results from the setting up of registers, although maintaining an up to date register is also labour intensive—electronic data linkage and data transfer can reduce these costs.

8   National Collation of Data held on Local Registers

If all health authorities collect comparable data it should be possible to aggregate this information at national level thereby facilitating the generation of comparative data, for example enabling comparisons between districts to be undertaken. Again, it is unlikely that this will happen unless electronic transfer of data is in place.

Using Population based Registers for Call/Recall

So far I have mainly concentrated on the use of population-based information systems in the future planning and development of diabetes services. However, population-based registers can also be used as call/recall systems to remind patients to attend for their annual review and to remind health professionals that the annual review is due. Even if reminders are not sent to all patients, patients who have not been reviewed in the previous year, or whose review is incomplete, can be identified so that they can be specifically targeted for further follow up. Alternatively, population-based registers can be used to invite patients to have their eyes examined as part of a district wide diabetic eye screening programme.

Conclusions

It is my personal opinion that:

1   Each provider should maintain a register of diabetic patients under their care which should be updated at least annually. All providers should be strongly encouraged to use the BDA/RCP Recommended Data Set for recording information about their diabetic patients.

2   All health authorities should maintain population-based diabetes information systems which should be updated at least annually. Ideally, such systems should be linked to the FHSA database to enable automatic updating for changes of name and/or address, movements out of the district and deaths.

3   All patients should know what data are being recorded on both provider-based diabetes registers and health authority based diabetes information systems—they should ideally be given a printed copy of the information being entered on to the register.

4   The NHS should facilitate the national aggregation of data.

2
Information
Technology

Overview

The potential for Information Technology in disease management registers is enormous, but care needs to be taken not to overburden General Practitioners with time-consuming and costly information gathering requirements. The principle must be that 'simple is best'. The extent of use of Information Technology in general practice varies, and the needs of all General Practitioners must be taken into account. The NHS Executive's Report of the Efficiency Scrutiny into Bureaucracy in General Practice otherwise referred to as *Patients not Paper,* includes significant information management and technology initiatives, which start the process of electronic exchange of data between General Practitioners and provider trusts. Issues such as security of data and Read codes are being addressed, and the scope for the eventual use of the NHSnet and NHSweb is set out. There is a vast amount of data already held in general practice, on different computer software systems. The joint Department of Health and Northern Regional Health Authority-funded *Morbidity Information Query and Export Syntax* (MIQUEST) project has been developed by Northumberland Family Health Services Authority. The main aim was to enable anonymised data to be collected and integrated from different GP systems to enable improvements in health care planning and commissioning in the context of a primary care led NHS. Work on this will be taken forward by another NHS Executive project called "Collection of Health Data from General Practice" subject to approval of the business case. Ways in which the new advances in information technology may revolutionise the work of the NHS are also discussed.

2.1 Electronic Records and Messages: Opportunities and Threats

Dr Tom Davies, General Practitioner and Chairman of the RCGP/GMSC
Computer Committee and the GP Group 1 Messaging Committee, Yaxley
Health Centre, Yaxley, Peterborough

Introduction

97% of the population in this country is registered with a general practitioner
(GP). As we move to a primary led NHS we have a wonderful opportunity.
Change has happened at a speed that would have been unthinkable just 10
years ago. We must ensure that we at last use technology to benefit the care
of the patient and the working conditions of the professional.

Long term surveillance of most medical care in this country is undertaken
by the primary health care team. Diabetes is but one example of a chronic
condition. Hypertension, asthma and epilepsy are also by and large looked
after within general practice. Out reach nurses, close working relationships
with local hospital departments and development of guidelines (shared by
local groups) have all helped drive the process. If general practice is to
continue to take on this work proper resources must be given to the team to
carry them out. Care in general practice shouldn't be chosen just on the
basis of costs. Quality matters and should be paid for.

Computerisation of general practice[1] has been one of the success stories of
the last 10 years (Table 1). Of the 79% of practices that were computerised,
90% were using their computers for clinical purposes, 29% fully, and a
further 19% partially but intending to go fully. 66% are entering clinical
data at some or all consultations. However it has to be acknowledged that
it is becoming apparent that there are problems with both how the data is
entered, and more specifically the quality of the clinical data being entered.
Too many practices saw computers as the solution to their problems, did
not properly plan, and continue to skim the surface and use them for the 3
'R's (Registration, recall and repeat prescribing.) By 1995 some 90%
practices are computerised and over 2000 are linked to FHSA's for transfer
of data. At the moment it is mostly used for administrative purposes
(registration and Items of service payments) and we must ensure that now
the technology is being put into place that it is used for clinical purposes as
well. Up till now, we have been constrained by much of the software. Doctors
and others need to say what we want and need, and not leave it to the
computer experts to give us what they think computers should do.

Table 1:   Number of Practices computerised

Year	%	No
1987	10	942
1988	19	1802
1989	28	1674
1990	47	4612
1991	63	6130
1992	71	6688
1993	79	7613
1993 DH Survey		

We must not forget from where we come and the problems we have with the present methods of recording information i.e. written notes, both in general practice and hospitals. In general practice we keep records for a variety of reasons, as a record of each encounter, but also as a database of information and a filing system for letters, reports, investigations etc. Bulk of the record and retrievability of information is a real problem. As we move to an electronic record we must decide whether the GP's record is to be a comprehensive archive record (with everything) or just a Primary Care Record[2]. (Tables 2a/b : summary of both types of GP record)

Table 2:   Which Type of GP Record?
after Ridsall Smith

Table 2a: Archive Record

Comprehensive
Hard to assess facts
Cumbersome
Medicolegally safe
Expensive
Bulky, takes space+

Table 2b: Primary care record

Only keep relevant records
Easy structured access
Brief easy recording
Medicoleg. vulnerable
Easy filing
Cheap

At the present time we really face a major disincentive to fully using computers because of the duplication required both entering data on the computer, and being required by our terms of service to keep proper written record. The Legitimisation of the Electronic record group have made recommendations that hopefully will soon be accepted. Obviously before one goes 'paperless' the systems must be safe and have adequate audit trails. Already it is estimated that some 10% of GPs who are computerised and using the computer for clinical recording have claimed to have gone paperless (or paperfree at the point of patient contact).

Problems of the Medical Record

Table 3 summarises the present problems with using written records for most of us. The situation will be very familiar. The benefits (and initial struggles) with the computerised record must always be compared with the inherent problems (and inefficiencies) of the system we are using at the moment. Notes are often missing, lost or not available, and this leads to the creation of temporary/ duplicate records. X-rays, investigations are all kept separately. Reports are not properly filed. The notes are often bulky, falling to bits and contain excess, duplicate and unnecessary information. Letters are not filed sequentially, and much time is lost going through the notes. Information from other hospitals is rarely acquired and accumulated. Handwriting is often illegible, with results difficult to view sequentially, and no graphical displays. There is a lack of consistency between departments / hospitals. Crucially important information (Allergies etc.) is easily lost.

Table 3   Problems with written records
after Stewart Orr

Problems of the Medical Record

- Locating the casenotes, daytime and out of hours
- Physical state of the casenotes
- Organisation of documents in the casenotes
- Organisation of information in the casenotes
- Wasteful effort
- Communications problems
- Administrative Problems
- Problems of access to related information
- General Medical problems

There are delays in receiving referrals, letters, summaries, prescribing information, etc. and often inaccurate and out of date information is used (GP's, addresses, admissions etc.). There is poor co-ordination between many departments/Primary care/Social Services Departments (SSDs). Inadequate follow up often arises from casenotes being removed to another location without being properly processed.

Data collection for audit is almost impossible. Decision support is impossible and action on guidelines/protocols difficult.

The opportunity we now have is to move to the fully electronic record. We must hurry and agree on the structure for all the professions to agree (The Multi-professional Working group on the core structure for communicating the personal health record is at this present time working out the basic details). In primary care all the team must use and add to the computerised record, and it must be flexible enough to output information in the way the nurse, dietician, dispenser, doctor and indeed the patient needs.

Table 4 highlights the IM & T Strategy. However there is a very simple paradox that we must address namely:–

> *Clinicians won't use computers until they are genuinely useful, and have full clinical information on them—Full information won't be on computers until clinicians use them!*

Table 4:   IM & T Strategy

- Information will be person based
- Systems should be integrated
- Information will be derived from operational systems
- Information will be secure and confidential
- Information will be shared across the NHS
- Information will be health based

The Electronic record does confer major benefits to patient care. Information that is relevant and comprehensive is immediately available at the appropriate places and times. Reduced clinical errors should occur (over come temptation to come to snap diagnosis) . Important information can be highlighted, (allergies etc.) which with paper is often buried and never seen! (on screen, instantly get the whole picture) and time should be saved chasing letters, results etc. Results should be instantly available. Target groups can be recalled, monitored and Decision Support is coming. Medical Audit can be supported and external resource usage, (pathology, referrals) monitored and compared with others. The electronic record supports teaching and CME and research, epidemiological monitoring.

I admit at the present rarely is the information electronically transmitted and much duplication, triplication takes place. The rule for the future should be:–

*Information entered on an NHS computer is only entered once.
If needed by other professionals this information should be
transmitted electronically*

Another benefit I have found is one that initially I feared the most, namely the presence of computer in the consulting room. It has actually led to a more open consulting style. Placing the terminal in full view of the patient encourages a full and open discussion, and areas of concern can be highlighted. The presence of multimedia programmes now can lead to clinicians showing all types of things to patients with improved patient involvement and education. Customised printouts can be provided for patients to take away, and in our practice put in their patient held records.

Table 5 summarises the benefits. The transmission must be more than simple E-mail, and the UN/EDIFACT message should be developed with all speed. Unfortunately at the present time to few of the profession seem to realise the benefits or the issues. Poor systems, concentrating on Administration data has jaundiced the mainstream clinicians view of computers.

Table 5:   The benefits of Electronic Links

Speed (avoid treating 'on spec')
Accurate
Structured - direct input to GP systems
Comprehensive
Avoids duplications
May be sent to many

In 1987 International Organisation for Standardisation (ISO) adopted EDI standard managed by United Nations (UN/EDIFACT and the NHSME EL (92) 34 adopted as NHS standard in 1992. EDIFACT has been used for 7 years in NHS starting with purchasing supplies and processing dental claims. In 1992 3 trial messages were developed in the Message Programme, namely GP-Pathology Links, GP-Radiology Links and GP-Hosp. Discharge/admission/death notifications. These messages were signed off by CIG in December 1994 and piloting is now occurring. Future message groups to be set up in the near future include Cervical Cytology, Accident and Emergency and Pharmacy.

I believe that the time is right and hope I have given a positive message, though I acknowledge there are some potential dangers/problems. The BMA/GMSC have major concerns with links, and wish for encryption for all messages. Obviously sensitive information must be protected and risk from deliberate attempts to sabotage or hacking possible. There are new dangers in the scale, quantity and distribution. The benefits for clinicians in ease of use and to see easily what is there applies to authorised users (for

---

other purposes) having sight of records of people they shouldn't be seeing.

The 4 control security levels to be used for the NWN project are :–
1 No connection to system. High sensitive e.g. AIDS Databases
2 Use of PAD (Personal Authentication Device)
3 Dial Back facility
4 Conventional password

Read Codes

Initially used in general practice, and recommended for use in the NHS by the JCG in 1988 it is now time for the NHS to properly and fully implement the Read Codes. The principles behind the classification are fully accepted. Namely that they facilitate clinical care, allow statistical analysis and allow transmission of data. General practitioners should be allowed to use Versions 4 and 5 with the terms they need for messaging before migrating to version 3 in the next two or three years.

References

1   Department of Health, "Computerisation in GP Practices." Survey prepared by Social Services (Gallup Poll) Ltd. (Department of Health, 1993)

2   Ridsall Smith: Personal Communication

3   Orr, S., "Integrated Clinical Workstation User Requirements (Acute Hospitals) Part B. Version 4." (1993) NHS Centre for Coding Classification, Woodgate, Loughborough.

4   Markwell, D., "Computerised Patient Records in General Practice—Guidelines for Good Practice." (1995) NHS Executive Performance Management Directorate

2.2 Registers and New Information Technology: Exploiting the Multi-Media World and Information Super-Highway

Ms P Hodgson, Information Management Group, NHS Executive, Leeds

Introduction

An NHS-wide electronic networking system (the "NHSnet") is at the centre of the NHS Information Management & Technology (IM&T) infrastructure. The core of the network system will be provided by British Telecom, largely through private finance. It is now available to the NHS.

The business case for NHSnet as approved by the Treasury was primarily based on the high volume "bread and butter" information flows across the NHS, such as electronic mail, exchange of contract information and supplies ordering. There is also a key requirement for links between General Practitioners and hospitals and General Practitioners and Health Authorities as the recent "Patients not Paper" report has confirmed.

As demand for networking facilities or "bandwidth" increases, British Telecom will simply "call down" the necessary resources. There is therefore no technical limit to the type of service available.

Running over the NHSnet will be Internet-type facilities called the NHSweb. The NHSweb is a collection of sites (an intranet rather than the Internet) sitting on NHSnet, each with their own NHSweb URL, offering information and services designed to meet the purposes of the NHS. Providers of NHSweb information and services will be drawn from within the NHS itself and from outside organisations. The NHSweb Directory will provide information about all information and services available on NHSweb and elsewhere which may be of interest and use to people in the NHS.

The potential of the network infrastructure is creating considerable interest. The NHS Executive's Information Management Group (IMG) has received a significant number of proposals from academia and industry offering to provide the NHS with a range of services.

The following are brief descriptions of the main types of service proposals and their potential to revolutionise the working of the NHS.

Telemedicine

At the simplest end of the spectrum, real time video links can be set up to enable General Practitioners and their patients to diagnose and discuss care plans with consultants in other locations. At the more complex end of the spectrum, keyhole surgery could be performed at a distance, with the aid of a real time video link, by an extremely specialised surgeon. Obviously these possibilities need to be carefully trialled before being made available. Nevertheless, it is already apparent that there is potential for re-engineering the way in which the NHS works.

Education

Access to video banks and decision support systems can facilitate continuing clinical education. Network Services will enable NHS staff to access the latest versions of text books or course material in electronic format. It will be possible electronically to broadcast lectures to students. Staff will be able to see operations performed in real time at locations remote from them (not only in the UK). The education, particularly the continuing education of healthcare professionals and other NHS staff could be transformed.

Knowledge Bases

By means of Network Services, all types of healthcare professionals including General Practitioners and Public Health specialists will be able to access the latest information on a vast range of material. The NHS Executive's Research and Development Information Strategy was created to ensure that the latest results from research work particularly from the Cochrane Centre were made quickly and easily available to the NHS. Knowledge bases of pharmaceutical products and information on outcome measures are just two examples of what could be made available.

Bulletin Boards and News Services

These have significant potential to improve the way information is communicated to NHS staff. Modern technology can also enable them to interact with these types of services to feedback views and order services.

The Information Management Group will provide an NHSnet directory to enable users to navigate easily around the services on the NHSnet.

Steps Taken to Date

Ministers have agreed that the quality of information available on the NHSnet should be left to the professions where they decm it necessary.

A "Networking Applications Advisory Group" has been established involving experts from the NHS and industry and the other home countries.

The Group is concerned with establishing mechanisms for dealing with proposals from suppliers and the NHS to provide application services to the NHS.

The Group has decided that some basic rules have to be determined for organisations offering to provide a Service on the NHSnet. These will cover the following:

- The requirements of the NHS-Wide Networking Security Code of Connection must be satisfied.
- Proposals for application services will be scrutinised by members of a Reference Group to ensure that any proposal is in line with current policy and to decide who shall have an entry in the directory.

Registers and the NHSNET

There are many registers available and some are being developed that can be made available over the NHSnet.

Registers are used in the health service to identify patients and other members of the population for healthcare delivery (for example in Patient Administration Systems, diabetes and asthma systems) and for a variety of health promotion, screening and preventive care services (for example child development, vaccination and immunisation, cervical and breast screening).

Each of these systems have been supported by their own patient registers but in future there will be the opportunity to use the Administrative Register. The Information Management Group is already developing an Administrative Register which strategically is likely to become the primary source of administrative information to which all other systems will interface and use to validate their data.

The NHS Administrative Registers will bring a number of key benefits:

- enabling more efficient care eg through reduction in failed appointments and improved accuracy in correspondence;
- aiding in the identification of special needs groups and contract planning;
- providing access to aggregate information for planning and analysis; and
- providing a means for health event linkage between systems.

IMG's role is to provide the infrastructure enabling these benefits. It will be up to individual purchasers and providers to exploit the combination of the NHSnet and the Administrative Register to realise the great opportunities provided by the power of technology.

The GP Scrutiny Review—"Patients Not Paper"

There are some significant Information Management & Technology initiatives in "Patients not Paper" which start the process of developing Electronic Data Interchange (EDI) messages between General Practitioners and Providers, (both acute and community health trusts). Clinical messages, such as referral and discharge letters and pathology laboratory requests and results, will be implemented in a number of "trailblazer" sites during 1996. Discussions will also take place on which other messages are also appropriate for EDI links, so continually reducing bureaucracy between General Practitioners and Providers.

"Patients not Paper" also covers a wide range of other EDI links, including General Practice Fundholders access to clearing house data; the production of electronic versions of the Red Book and Drug Tariff; public health access to General Practice clinical data for epidemiological purposes; and further General Practice/FHSA administrative links, including data from the cervical cytology recall scheme. Improved training programmes for clinicians in information and IT are also planned as part of IMG's initiatives.

The "Patients not Paper" clinical messages have been agreed with the professions concerned and the aims of the "Patients not Paper" Programme is to work with all parties in the NHS, (General Practitioners, Commissioners, Providers and Regional Offices), and the various computer suppliers, in order to move the NHS into an IM&T environment. The ultimate aim is to use IM&T solutions to improve patient care and the effectiveness of the NHS in delivering patient care.

2.3 Sharing General Practice Data
Formerly The Continuous Collection of Health Data from GP Systems

Andrew Kent, Corporate Affairs Directorate, Information Management Group, NHS Executive, Leeds

Dave Smith, Corporate Affairs Directorate, Information Management Group, NHS Executive, Leeds

Introduction

Everyone is aware that there is a vast amount of data held by general practitioners (GPs) in a wide range of systems some of which may be used locally for a variety of reasons. However this is an untapped resource as there is an increasing interest in the potential value of information collected by GPs. This information is of growing importance not only to GPs but also to health authorities, public health departments, medical audit groups and research projects. But why should we use the data and how can it be accessed and then used? The data collected is of course for a specific purpose but many GPs do not have the facilities to have the data analysed. This is where the sharing of the data (suitably anonymised) by say health authorities (HAs) can provide an improved service particularly to assist effective purchasing and the better use of resources in the delivery of patient care.

A major study was undertaken in 1993 into the feasibility and desirability of some form of national scheme for the regular collection and analysis of health data from general practice. Its conclusions are still considered to be relevant, although the scope of the project needs to be reviewed in the light of changes that have taken placed over the last two years, particularly the expanding role of GPs both as purchasers and providers.

The study identified an impressive list of information requirements of the centre and the NHS that could be met in whole or part by GP health data. Information derived from GP data will assist with health needs assessment, resource planning, target monitoring, assessment of service effectiveness, and in providing indications of outcomes. The study recommended that local collection schemes be established by health authorities working in conjunction with local GP representative groups, and that central information needs would be met by extracting data from local schemes into a separate central analysis and reporting facility. This arrangement would be implemented in a phased manner whereby the numbers of contributors and local schemes, and the scope of the data collected, would build over a period of five or six years. The first year of operation would be in the form of a pilot with six local schemes and about 200 practices in total. The first year scheme would be designed to test the software and procedures, and to ensure that the information produced could be put to practical use.

There have been and are several local collection schemes run by NHS organisations. However, most are still concentrating on collection methods and resolving data quality problems, and there is a shortage of hard evidence for the beneficial use of information derived from GP health data.

The systematic collection of GP data direct from computer systems would not involve practices in significant additional effort, although they would have to be prepared to comply with guidelines and minimum standards on data recording, that would be developed as part of the introduction of the scheme. This is necessary to ensure that the resultant information is credible and comparable.

The estimated running costs were sensitive to assumptions about payments to GPs, which seemed difficult to avoid altogether in the early stages, but could probably be reduced or eliminated over time as higher standards of data recording become the norm. In general, the costs appeared reasonable in relation to the potential uses of information that could be derived and the benefits from such use. Setting up a national framework would also have the effect of avoiding costs that would otherwise almost certainly be borne by individual health authorities.

Design and development work was halted in late 1993 when DH acquired the ex-VAMP database (now called the GP Research Database (GPRD)) of patient health event data. It has over 550 contributing practices covering 6.5% of the population, and it was thought that it might represent an alternative to setting up a new NHS collection scheme. Evaluation studies conducted during 1994 concluded that the GPRD in its current form could meet only a small proportion of the GP-related information requirements of DH and the NHS.

An example of a local initiative is MIQUEST which stands for **Morbidity Information QUery and Export SynTax.** This was a project jointly funded by the Department and the then Northern RHA and was developed at Northumberland FHSA. The high level definition is 'to facilitate the collection of health data from different GP computer systems by defining a Health Query Language (HQL)'. The HQL consists of two parts: a patient centred dictionary and a formally specified query language. It is capable of expressing the many current and potential requirements for extraction of data held on different GP systems. As well a being a query language for use by external enquirers HQL also provides a greater level of reporting functionality than is available in most GP computer systems.

Now if you are not of a technical disposition this basically means that:

- a range of query styles can be used by say a HA to identify particular areas of interest.
- the query is then passed to the GP system for consideration and approval to release the information
- the approved data is provided in an requested (standard) format taking account of the analysis required. for example 'count diabetic patients by type of diabetes, ages etc etc.

So where are we now? The project has been reactivated. The end products of the first phase of work have been defined as a detailed implementation plan and a business case. This will involve drawing up realistic, costed plans for at least two options with different scope and/or development/ technical approaches. Guidance from the Project Board will be sought on which options to pursue.

Work currently being undertaken which will feed into the implementation plan and business case will include:

- finalising the statements of business needs and information requirements.
- prioritising information requirements and evaluating potential benefits.
- identifying and exploring any issues that might prevent successful implementation of the recommended scheme, including data confidentiality and legitimate uses of GP data;
- identifying and assessing technical options including data flows and technical architecture, and recommending the best approach;
- investigating whether special system development effort can be avoided by the use of software already in use by such as GPRD and MIQUEST.
- use of Read codes;

So what next. Firstly we do not believe that we have all the answers, in fact we are not sure if we know what all the questions are that we should be asking. Basically we do not want to reinvent wheels but work with initiatives that are already happening. The advantage of this method is that a lot of good points will already start to emerge and that mistakes will have happened and started to be overcome. It may prove that none of the local systems have the capability for transforming into a national system but on the other hand there may be one that is the answer to all our prayers.

We do not aim to be exclusive or claim all the credit and if there is anything happening out there that may provide positive input to our project then we want to know about it. Also if there is anything in the work that we are doing that can be of use to others then we are happy to share that too.

Details of MIQUEST are already available. The material, both paper and electronic, is quite extensive so order forms are available for you to select what is most appropriate for your area of interest.

2.4 Integrated Clinical Workstation: Short Report of a Demonstration

Dr Ian Bowns, Information Management Group, NHS Executive, Leeds
Dr Rob Hampton, NHS Centre for Coding and Classification, Woodgate, Loughborough

A computerised simulation intended to help professional colleagues see how information management and technology can in the future contribute to seamless clinical care and assist in the maintenance of disease registers was demonstrated.

The simulation showed how the projects within the NHS Information Management and Technology Strategy (NHS IM&T Strategy), such as NHS Wide Networking, will support multi-disciplinary disease management across health care settings.

The simulation is based around an imaginary patient with diabetes, who had previously had a leg amputated because of complications of the disease, first sees a community nurse. The nurse undertakes a clinical history and examination, and makes an electronic record of the consultation, including a video showing the patient's walking difficulties. The nurse then makes an electronic referral to the general practitioner.

The general practitioner (GP) receives the electronic referral, sees the patient and reviews the control of the diabetes. Use is made of clinical protocol, a drug formulary, and pictures in a medical library are used to assist the diagnosis of an unusual rash. All of these services are available via the computer, rather than as documents.

Having altered the dose of drugs used to control the diabetes, the GP refers the patient to a consultant dermatologist. A second referral is made to the local Appliance Centre to adjust the patient's artificial leg which will reduce his walking difficulties. Both referrals use electronic mail.

Throughout the demonstration, use is made of the computer mouse, or "point and click" technology, to simplify the rapid recording of structured data with minimal interference to the consultation, reducing the need for the keyboard.

Whilst this is a simulation and not a genuine system, the technologies to undertake each particular task is now available. Electronic mail is in widespread use, powerful personal computers now cost little more than

£1,000, and video recording and conferencing equipment is now in use in commerce and the NHS. The fulfilment of the NHS IM&T Strategy aims to provide the communications and standards infrastructure for clinical information systems to live up to this vision.

3
Diabetes Registers

Overview

The case for the use of registers as an aid to improving the quality of care delivered to people with diabetes is reviewed in this paper. It also gives a personal view point of the more important characteristics of diabetes registers, in particular the dataset. Bearing in mind that the burden of collecting most of this data will fall on the General Practitioner, and mindful of the NHS Executive's Report of the Efficiency Scrutiny into Bureaucracy in General Practice [Ref: Leeds NHS Executive 1995], otherwise referred to as *Patients not Paper,* the dataset should be **simple** and provide information which is useful for the management of the person with diabetes. For comparative purposes across the district the dataset should be comparable.

3.1 The Nature of Registers in Diabetes Care: A Personal View of a Consultant Diabetologist

Professor Philip Home, Department of Medicine, Freeman Diabetes Service, University of Newcastle upon Tyne, Newcastle

Introduction

The concept of using, as an aid to quality health care delivery, some kind of register of people with known diabetes mellitus, is not new. Indeed in the UK one of the two pioneer districts of a population-based diabetes health care system developed a computerized record of all people in its care system from its earlier days[1,2]. Other secondary care clinical services have also found comprehensive diabetes registers to be a foundation of optimal diabetes care, and again the history of these implementations now stretches back some 15 years[3,4].

The stimulus to such ideas is multifactorial, but contains a number of facets which are relevant to current implementations of diabetes registers, and are therefore worth consideration here:–

- there are large numbers of people with diabetes in any population (~2 %), all needing continuing health care;
- the condition is progressive both in its metabolic pathogenesis and in the development of the so-called late complications; management must therefore be continual and active[5];
- non-insulin-dependent diabetes (in contrast to Type 1 (insulin-dependent) diabetes which is a pure hormone deficiency disease) is a complicated condition requiring attention to many facets of management[6];
- most continuing management of diabetes is preventative care (attention to blood glucose and blood lipid control, smoking, blood pressure, and the like), requiring professionals to initiate care rather than to respond to patient symptoms;
- both preventative care and surveillance for complications are effective and cheap, compared to the impact and costs of treatment of the eye, heart, renal and foot complications when they develop;
- care has always been provided in both the primary and secondary sectors, but the pattern of provision of that care varies widely according to professional skills and interest.

There is however a more contemporary history to diabetes registers, and this has had major consequences for their current structure, and poses important limitations on the nature of registers that should now be implemented in Europe. In 1989, under the auspices of the European Region of the World Health Organization (WHO) and the International Diabetes Federation (IDF) –the latter representing patient associations–, representatives of governments, patients, professionals and others, came together at St Vincent (Italy) to formulate the programme now generally known as the St Vincent Declaration Initiative[7]. Governments subsequently endorsed this at a regional World Health Assembly. One of the targets of the Declaration was the " . . . establishment of monitoring systems . . . for quality assurance . . . ". Subsequently considerable time and effort has been devoted to developing an international standard for data collection and data exchange (the DiabCare initiative[8]), and it is consequently important that registers conform to this standard.

In the UK the parallel (and compatible) initiative has primarily been devoted to the development of a UK recommended diabetes dataset[9,10], which has now been adopted by most of the diabetes-specific software packages. The importance of this being firmly grounded in routine diabetes practice, and the development of entry level reduced datasets[11], are discussed below and in other articles in this report. Standards are also available for data analysis[9].

Failures of Routine Diabetes Care

To be justified on both health and economic grounds, any development in health care delivery must clearly meet a need and have significant impact on it. In diabetes care it is well recognized that there are significant failures in our present attempts to deliver an adequate (not necessarily optimal) level of care to all those with the condition[12]. This is unacceptable in a condition in which there is considerable evidence that morbidity can be substantially reduced by attention to preventative measures, and in particular optimization of blood glucose and blood lipid control, reduction in prevalence of smoking, control of blood pressure, simple foot care measures to prevent ulceration and amputation, surveillance for sight-threatening eye damage, and aspirin for ischaemic heart disease[13-17]. Inspection of the actual delivery of care suggests that such failures have their basis in the problems that professionals have in paying repeated attention to health care problems which are not symptomatic, in particular, as in non-insulin-dependent diabetes, where a number of these cluster together. Accordingly one sees a failure to emphasize preventative care, a failure to screen for early complications and risk factors, and poor levels of communication and education to encourage patient self-care. These findings are nearly always associated with poor (unstructured) record systems, and care which is not protocol guided.

The Clinical Services Advisory Group (Diabetes) noted that lack of information systems was a characteristic of Health Districts with deficiencies in the provision of diabetes care, and that this together with a low awareness of the health care and economic impact of diabetes, led to relative under-resourcing of such care[18]. The use of information systems is clearly easily integrated into a system of structured record keeping, targets for metabolic and other intermediate health outputs, and use of the data to inform the quality assurance process. Furthermore the performance of annual surveillance for detection of the development of treatable complications is now enshrined in many published protocols and guidelines for diabetes care[19,6], including those espousing patients rights to care[20,21], and information systems can provide the opportunity for the implementation of recall systems to support such surveillance.

The Role of Registers in Diabetes Care

It will already be clear that the term 'register', when used in the sense of a compilation of cases and their characteristics, leads to a misunderstanding of what is needed in diabetes care. The two major factors which determine that divergence are the progressive nature of the continuing condition[5], and as a result the changing characteristics, and the use of the information for quality assurance and recall purposes. The quality assurance function further implies local analysis and feedback of confidential data, further divorcing the diabetes register from the health statistics approach.

The major roles which diabetes registers have been devised to serve are then:–

1   *Quality assurance*

    Based on biomedical datasets endorsed by the medical profession and already incorporated in all the major diabetes software packages, this allows review of achievements by comparison to targets and other services of process measures (such as eye screening), true health outcomes (such as limb amputation), risk factor management (such as smoking and blood pressure control), and intermediate outcomes (such as achieved blood glucose and blood lipid control)[9.]

    Useful reports can be prepared on the basis of as few as 50 people with diabetes (and thus a small general practice) for some process measures and achieved blood glucose control. At the other end of the spectrum advances in diabetes care have meant that the incidence of some of the adverse late complications such as blindness and renal failure is becoming quite low where care is more optimal, necessitating collation of data from all local care sites before the numbers become meaningful.

2   *Health care recall and surveillance*

    Recall for surveillance for treatable complications can usefully be integrated with quality assurance systems, particularly as the data collected as a result of surveillance (for example the process of eye screening and the presence or absence of sight-threatening retinopathy), are identical to those included within the recommended datasets. Recall systems are important for two reasons:–

a   eye screening for retinopathy is regarded by many general practitioners as the major barrier to their confidence in running practice diabetes services; an eye recall system can be linked to a retinal screening programme using a retinal camera, optometrists, or opthalmoscopists;

b   annual recall serves as a catch all to ensure not only that necessary complication surveillance should occur[23], but also that metabolic control and arterial risk factors have been optimized as far as is possible; some services have integrated patient education into their annual review system[24].

3   Needs assessment

There remains an urgent need for reliable data to inform needs assessment about people with diabetes, particularly for those involved in commissioning care. This partly relates to differences in the prevalence of diabetes itself, as it is known to be strongly influenced (increased prevalence) in particular by the ethnic mix of populations, and independently of this by social deprivation[25]. The importance of these issues is best illustrated by noting that health care resource consumption as a result of diabetes is around 5 % of the total health budget, and that either of those factors could easily double this.

The datasets devised for recall and quality assurance are suitable for needs assessment, covering as they do data items which allow assessment of the number of people with the different types of diabetes, age structure, prevalence of complications and adverse outcomes requiring additional medical resources, and the distribution of people with diabetes by sites of care. It would be logical that individual data could easily be used to help prompt the care of people with diabetes as to the care site most appropriate to their needs. As yet there is no published record of this having been done.

Managers consulted in NHS research and development priority setting exercises have been amongst the groups who have recognised the development and deployment of such information systems as the first priority in the diabetes care area. Published information is now available for example which illustrates the extent of the needed expansion of both primary and secondary care sectors, when a district-wide diabetes care system is implemented[26].

Characteristics of the Required Registers

In this section, for the sake of brevity, two necessary aspects of the characteristics of diabetes registers will be discussed together. The first aspect concerns the characteristics of any information system (and its implementation) being commissioned to support diabetes care. At the same time some of the considerations which have guided the development of these ideas and tools will be discussed.

1   The dataset used by the information system must be compatible with the UK recommended dataset in use in other systems. Ideally the dataset should be identical with the UK dataset[9,10], although in principle as long as an export function using the same dataset structure is available, then it will still be possible to collate data from different sources both for comparison of the care achieved (on a confidential basis) and for aggregation for needs assessment purposes. The UK dataset is itself compatible with the European DiabCare dataset[27].

Considerable care in constructing the UK dataset has gone into ensuring that it is based on information already collected in any adequate diabetes care system, and therefore that it does not require or consume extra medical resources beyond those of routine clinical care[9]. For optimal data abstraction however (as well as optimal care) a structured care record is also needed, whether as part of a normal medical record or specific diabetes record card. The UK dataset includes precise definitions of the content of each data-field (for example male erectile impotence such as to obviate the possibility of vaginal penetration); these are also necessary if data is to be compiled from multiple sites of care.

Additionally the dataset has a hierarchical structure, which allows it to be adopted in sites of care where the detail of diabetes records is presently less than generally recommended, and where the approach to the full dataset might be a barrier to its implementation. Thus in addition to the recommended dataset there are entry and intermediate level datasets compatible with the main dataset[11].

2   Quality assurance analytical software should be provided as part of the package. This is important if providers of data are to obtain any feedback from the information they provide. At its simplest this will include an analysis of the processes actually performed at any site of care, together with assessments of the numbers of patients with particular complications, and the achievements in respect of metabolic outcomes and risk factor management[9].

Both in the UK and in Europe packages are being developed to allow comparison of achieved results in key areas with other services, mainly

---

using benchmarking software. It is presently a normal understanding that only the site of care providing data should be able to identify itself.

3   A recall facility for Annual Review and eye screening should be provided. In some services these functions are combined, but in others they may be provided as separate functions[24], and it may be useful to separate the recall system into two. Where the information system is provided for a locality then it will most sensibly operate on the same basis as the more familiar cervical screening systems, but with pre-notification to a nominated responsible clinician for each individual patient. Such a system is reliant on an up to date demographic register, and it may be that this will be best provided by a link between the diabetes system and the Family Health Services Authority main register.

4   As it is envisaged that the largest possible functional unit for diabetes registers will be a population basis of around 500 000, it will always be the case that there will be a need for provision of data downloads so that comparisons can be made between localities in terms of achieved care. Planning for such a national facility is already underway. It seems likely that any such download will have to be in the structure of the UK recommended dataset, either in dBase or ASCII format.

5   Those commissioning diabetes registers need also be aware of the need to maintain flexibility so that they can take advantage of further developments in the use of diabetes datasets to promote optimal diabetes care as they become available. Some of those developments (benchmarking software, needs assessment software, software for identification of optimal site of care) have been referred to already. Other simple and obvious ideas include software to inform professionals of the economic consequences of their clinical decisions, and software to support and prompt simple clinical decision making such as timing, dosage, and drug choice for anti-hypertensive treatment.

More particularly a small extension to the recommended dataset can allow it to form the basis of an electronic patient record, and it would seem likely that this could provide the basis of an integrated care record, that is a single record for each individual completed independent of care site.

It would be inappropriate to delay the deployment of a quality assurance, needs assessment, and recall system because of potential developments of this type, which are likely to be unending. However building such modules into an existing system can be expensive, and it would therefore seem sensible at present either to establish a population-based register separate from any clinical information system (but able to communicate with any such system), or to ensure that the data structure used is such that it can be addressed by any new software package subsequently implemented on the same hardware (or with electronic access to it). In practical terms both these options imply the use of the recommended dataset.

Practical Experience of Diabetes Registers

It is not intended here to review experience to date with the type of diabetes register discussed above. The functioning and implementation of some example systems is discussed elsewhere in this report.

It is perhaps worth noting however that examples of implementation of diabetes information systems, both pre-dating the UK dataset and more recently using it, are available on a population basis (and therefore involving primary health care) from a number of sites in the UK. Indeed the concepts developed under the St Vincent Declaration Initiative have of course been adopted in a number of European countries, notably in France where the Assistance Publique is now promoting national implementation following a widespread trial in Paris, and in primary health care in Portugal.

It does not seem then that questions of practicality should delay more widespread implementation of diabetes registers in the UK, although care must be taken to address issues of data ownership, confidentiality, and the means of comprehensive data collection, as part of any implementation process.

References

1 Hill, R. D., "Diabetes and the computer." *Practical Diabetes* 3 (1986), 235–237, 290–297

2 Hill, R., "Community services for diabetics in the Poole area." *British Medical Journal* i (1976),1137–1139

3 Jones, R. B., Hedley, A. J., "A computer in the diabetic clinic." *Practical Diabetes* 3 (1986), 295–296

4 Williams, C. D., Harvey, F. E., Sonksen, P.H., "A role for computers in diabetes care?" *Diabetic Medicine* 5 (1988), 177–199

5 *United Kingdom Prospective Diabetes Study Group.* United Kingdom prospective diabetes study (UKPDS) 13: "relative efficacy of randomly allocated diet, sulphonylurea, insulin or metformin in patients with newly diagnosed non-insulin dependent diabetes followed for three years." *British Medical Journal* (1995); 310: 83–88

6 *European NIDDM Policy Group.* "A desk-top guide for the management of non-insulin-dependent diabetes mellitus (NIDDM)." *Diabetic Medicine* 11 (1994), 899–909

7 *World Health Organisation (Europe) and International Diabetes Federation (Europe).* "Diabetes care and research in Europe: the St Vincent declaration." *Diabetic Medicine* 7 (1990), 360–360

8 Piwernetz, K., Home, P. D., Snorgaard, O., Antsiferov, M., Staehr-Johansen, K., Krans, M., *for the DiabCare Monitoring Group of the St Vincent Declaration Steering Committee.* "Monitoring the targets of the St Vincent declaration and the implementation of quality management in diabetes care: the DiabCare initiative." *Diabetic Medicine* 10 (1993), 371–377

9 Wilson, A. E., Home, P.D., *for the Diabetes Audit Working Group of the Research Unit of the Royal College of Physicians and the British Diabetic Association.* "A dataset to allow exchange of information for monitoring continuing diabetes care." *Diabetic Medicine* 10 (1993), 378–390

10 Vaughan, N. J. A., Home, P. D., *for the Diabetes Audit Working Group of the Research Unit of the Royal College of Physicians and the British Diabetic Association.* "The UK diabetes dataset." *Diabetic Medicine* 12 (1995), 717–722

11 Alexander, W., Bradshaw, C., Gadsby, R., Home, P. D., Kopelman, P., MacKinnon, M., et al. "An approach to manageable datasets in diabetes care." *Diabetic Medicine* 11 (1994), 806–811

12 Williams, D. R. R., Munroe, C., Hospedales, C.J., Greenwood, R. H., "A three-year evaluation of the quality of diabetes care in the Norwich community care scheme." *Diabetic Medicine* 7 (1990), 74–79

13 *The DCCT Research Group.* "The diabetes control and complications trial (DCCT): The effect of intensive diabetes treatment on the effect of iontensive diabetes treatment on the development and progression of long-term complications in IDDM." *New England Journal of Medicine* 329 (1993), 977–986

14 Stewart, M. W., Laker, M. F., "Triglycerides in diabetes: a time for action?" *Diabetic Medicine* 11 (1994), 725–727

15 Neilsen, F. S., Rossing, P., Gall, M., Skott, P., Smidt, U. M., Parving, H., "Impact of lisinopril and atenolol on kidney function in hypertensive NIDDM subjects with diabetic nephropathy." *Diabetes* 43 (1994), 1108–1113

16 Day, J. L., "Patient education: how may recurrence be prevented?" in Connor, H., Boulton, A. J. M., Ward, J. D., (ed): The foot in diabetes. (Chichester Wiley, 1987), 135–143

17 Sculpher, M., Buxton, M. J., Ferguson, B. A., Humphreys, J. E., Altman, J. F. B., Spiegelhalter, D. J., et al. "A relative cost-effectiveness analysis of different methods of screening for diabetic retinopathy." *Diabetic Medicine* (1991), 644–650

18 *Clinical Standards Advisory Group.* "Standards of clinical care for people with diabetes." (HMSO, 1994)

19 *European IDDM Policy Group.* "Consensus guidelines for the management of insulin-dependent (Type 1) diabetes." *Diabetic Medicine* 10 (1993), 990–1005

20 *British Diabetic Association.* "Diabetes care what you should expect." (British Diabetic Association, 1993)

21 *International Diabetes Federation (Europe) and World Health Organization (Europe).* "The European Patients' Charter." *Diabetic Medicine* 8 (1991), 782–783

22 Williams, D. R. R., Home, P. D., *and members of a Working Group of the Research Unit of the Royal College of Physicians and the British Diabetic Association.* "A proposal for continuing audit of diabetes services." *Diabetic Medicine* 9 (1992), 759–764

23 Hurwitz, B., Goodman, C., Yudkin, J., "Prompting the clinical care of non-insulin-dependent (type II) diabetic patients in an inner city area: one model of community care." *British Medical Journal* 306 (1993), 624–630

24 *North Tyneside Diabetes Team.* "The diabetes annual review as an educational tool: assessment and learning integrated with care, screening and audit." *Diabetic Medicine* 9, (1992), 389–394

25 King, H., Zimmet, P.. "Trends in the prevalence and incidence of diabetes: non-insulin-dependent diabetes." *World Health Statistics Quarterly* 41 (1988), 190–196

26 Whitford, D. L., Southern, A. J., Braid, E., Roberts, S. H., "Comprehensive diabetes care in North Tyneside." *Diabetic Medicine* 12 (1995), 691–695

27 *DIABCARE Working Group.* "Monitoring instruments for improving the quality of diabetes care." In, Krans, H. M.J., Porta, M., Keen, H., Staehr Johansen, K., (ed): Diabetes care in Europe: the St Vincent Declaration action programme. (World Health Organization, 1995), 49–61

4
Personal Experiences

Overview

Diabetes registers in hospitals have been developed by enthusiastic diabetologists in a number of locations. Working with General Practitioners in the area, such registers are built up and maintained by a combination of outreach work gathering information in general practices themselves, and by patient interview during their visits to the hospital clinic. These may be developed into 'population-based' registers, but in some areas it may not be possible to capture data on *all* people with diabetes in the district health authority area because a number of diabetes clinics may exist each with their own register. Hospital-based registers are often much more sophisticated than those found in primary care settings, reflecting the specialist knowledge and expertise concentrated in the hospital clinic and the fact that such data are used for research purposes in addition to clinical management. It would be unreasonable to expect such a level of sophistication of General Practitioners, nor would it be necessary for strictly clinical management purposes. The location of a district population-based register in a hospital setting poses problems since the district health authority is ultimately responsible for the security and integrity of the data it would contain. District health authorities will use such data in making strategic decisions involving the allocation of resources between competing priorities. Districts should therefore be the first to be aware of what the aggregated and anonymised district data reveals about the health of their local population, and the effectiveness of care programmes. The way forward may well be for district health authorities themselves to take on responsibility for harnessing all data in the district, whether held in primary care or hospitals, and for analysing aggregated data before making it public.

It is for health authorities to decide whether they wish to make the necessary investment to establish and maintain such registers, the priority such an initiative would have, and the location of the register. District health authorities who set up district registers are responsible for the security and confidentiality of the data contained in such registers and should ensure that local arrangements make this clear. It is important to note that, in accordance with Departmental guidance (HSG(96)18), if anonymised information is sufficient for a particular purpose, identifiable data should be omitted wherever possible [ref is para 4.5]. Steps should therefore be taken to ensure that only anonymised aggregated data are sent to health authorities who are responsible for determining how such data may be used, including whether transfer to a third party is necessary.

Where an individual hospital provider is contracted to maintain a district register on behalf of the health authority, in addition to the security and confidentiality issues mentioned above, care should also be taken to ensure that:

- the health authority remains responsible for determining how data may be used;

- the data is truly population-based; and

- the dataset is simple and comparable across the district.

4.1 Personal Experience with a District Population Diabetic Register Located in General Practice

Dr Nick Cheales, General Practitioner, Paddock Wood, Kent

Dr Alistair Howitt, General Practitioner, Tonbridge, Kent

Introduction

In considering the management of patients with chronic diseases an accurate, well maintained register is a prerequisite to providing comprehensive and co-ordinated care[1]. The recent shifts in service provision from secondary to primary care, mean that more patients than ever receive much or all of their care within general practice. For many conditions, including diabetes, any population based register will need to include information obtained from general practice if it hopes to be comprehensive in its coverage.

In the past, studies have suggested that general practitioners (GPs) had difficulty in identifying patients and producing accurate data about them[2,3]. Is there any reason to alter this pessimistic view of the ability of general practice to contribute to population based registers?

The last few years have seen many disparate factors result in a radical change in the range and scope of information systems within general practice. Computerisation has developed at a rapid pace, the 1990 contract and amendments in 1993 to the regulations for chronic disease management clinics have required much enhanced information systems. Fundholding and locality commissioning have pushed general practice to the forefront of planning health care provision and required more detailed practice activity data. Audit within general practice has been increasingly used to inform and enhance the development of services provided.

We would like to relate our experience of producing a district diabetes register entirely from general practice information and then consider the factors that might motivate general practitioners and their teams to contribute to population based registers.

Tunbridge Wells District GP Diabetic Audit

In 1991 a group of 6 local GPs joined together to form a district general practitioner audit group. After discussing with local practices what they would like to audit, we agreed to attempt to organise a district wide diabetes audit.

It was agreed that practices would identify their diabetic patients as best as they could. Some practices had well established diabetic registers but the majority did not. Meanwhile, the audit group discussed with practices what aspects of diabetic care they wanted and thought feasible to audit. Additional advice was taken from hospital specialists on what they thought should be included and help was obtained from other groups attempting similar tasks elsewhere.

A single page questionnaire was used (see fig.1) and completed by the practice for every diabetic patient they identified. Completed questionnaires were returned to the audit group and the data processed using Epi-Info, a public domain software package originally devised for epidemiologists. In return for their hard work practices were sent a comprehensive report on their diabetic patients. Practices were also sent a district report based on non-attributable pooled data so that they could compare their performance with others. Follow up educational meetings were organised around the district.

TUNBRIDGE WELLS AUDIT GROUP DIABETIC AUDIT 1992–3

1 GP NAME _____
2 PATIENT SURNAME _____
3 PATIENT FIRST NAME _____
4 SEX: MALE / FEMALE
5 DATE OF BIRTH ____ / ____ / ____

6 YEAR OF DIAGNOSIS _____
7 TYPE OF CARE HOSPITAL
                 PRACTICE CLINIC
                 SHARED
                 UNSTRUCTURED
8 HOSPTIAL ATTENDED _____
9 HOSPITAL NUMBER _____
10 CURRENT TREATMENT INSULIN
                      TABLETS
                      DIET ONLY

11 HEIGHT _____ Metres
12 WEIGHT _____ Kg (in last year)

13 BLOOD PRESSURE   Y N   SYSTOLIC _____ mmHg
                             DIASTOLIC _____ mmHg
                             HYPERTENSION BEING TREATED Y / N

14 FOOT EXAMINATION   Y N
15 VISUAL ACTIVITY   Y N
16 VISUALIZATION OF FUNDI Y N
17 BLOOD SUGAR   Y N   Value _____ mmol/L   ONLY RECORD
18 GLYOCSYLATED Hb   Y N   Value _____ %   VALUE
19 CREATININE   Y N   Value _____ mmol/L   'N' ANSWERS 'Y'
20 PROTEINURIA   Y N   Absent/Present
21 CHOLESTEROL In last five years   Y N _____ Value   mmol/L
        Y=RECORDED IN THE LAST 12 MONTHS
        N=NO RECORDING IN THE LAST 12 MONTHS

22 SMOKING HISTORY   NOT RECORDED   NON SMOKER   SMOKER
   (Cigarettes)
                NUMBER OF CIGARETTES SMOKED _____ PER DAY

23 AMPUTATION Y / N   24 MYOCARDIAL INFARCTION Y / N   25 STROKE   Y / N
   (Diabetes related) T   T   T
26 DIALYSIS OR Y / N 27 REG BLIND OR PARTIALLY Y / N 28 RETINOPATHY Y / N
   TRANSPLANT   T   SIGHTED   T   (needing referral) T

Figure 1

We succeeded in enlisting the support of 41 of the 43 practices who use the local district hospital in which the group is based. The audit ran in its first cycle from 1992-1993, with data collection being completed within 6 months. It is worth noting that practices received no funding for their work and the audit took place before the introduction of chronic disease management (CDM) regulations relating to diabetes and asthma care.

The practices identified 2,574 diabetic patients giving a prevalence of 1.18%[4]. Other recent surveys using a variety of information sources produced very similar prevalences (Table 1). That two well conducted large-scale surveys (in Islington and Poole) produced prevalence rates similar to and less than the rate we achieved suggests that our method was at least as effective as other methods.

Table 1: Prevalence of diabetes

Location	Year	Number of patients	Prevalence (%)	Methods used to identify patients
Tunbridge Wells	1993	2574	1.18	General practice registers
Islington	1992	4674	1.17	General practice and hospital registers and PPA* returns
Trowbridge	1992	405	1.31	General practice and hospital registers
Powys	1989	469	1.01	General practice registers
Poole	1988	917	1.01	General practice and hospital registers
Oxford	1987	431	1.08	Hospital registers and postal questionnaires
Southall (Europeans)	1985	324	1.20	House to house

*PPA = Prescription Pricing Authority

Discussion

This was many practices first attempt at forming a diabetes register. Since this first attempt practices have been required to maintain a diabetic register under CDM regulations. Information collated from practice reports by Kent FHSA in 1994 suggests considerable improvement in the identification of diabetic patients with a prevalence for diabetes of 1.7%. (Clinical directorate, Kent Family Health Services Authority, personal communication)

Validity of the Data

If practices can identify their diabetic patients can they also provide valid data on them? This is of vital importance if such data are to be utilised within a population based register. In an attempt to answer this question we compared our data culled from 41 separate practices with data produced in published epidemiological surveys[4]. In comparing: current age, duration of diabetes, sex distribution, method of treatment, differences in glycosylated haemoglobin between treatment types and prevalence of complications, we found no significant differences between our data and that produced in a more rigorously controlled fashion from other sources.

Potential uses of the Data

The aim of our project was to facilitate a district wide general practice diabetes audit. It was not within our remit to produce a fully-fledged district diabetic register capable of call and recall. However, our experience in Tunbridge Wells suggests that general practice has the potential to contribute valuable information to population based registers.

What will Motivate General Practice to Collaborate with Population Based Registers?

Currently there is a strong sense of data/paper overload amongst general practitioners, a sentiment recognised in the recent high level government initiative to reduce paper work within public services. Scepticism of yet more paperwork and useless information will need to be overcome if general practice is to become actively involved in any given population based register.

Recently there has been much interest in the development of clinical guidelines and there is a growing body of literature on the factors that influence the effectiveness of guidelines[5][6][7]. We would suggest that there is considerable overlap between these factors and those that may influence the effective implementation of a population based register. A few key questions need to be considered:–

(i) Who will benefit from the register?

Clear and tangible benefits need to be demonstrated from the outset. By contributing data to the register, benefits must accrue to the patients concerned and to the practice that is attempting to deliver the necessary health care. Current recommendations for optimal diabetic care emphasise the importance of screening for complications and tighter glycaemic control [8][9]. A register that helps a practice with call and recall procedures and highlights defaulters will clearly be of benefit. Equally a register that helps co-ordinate care between different agencies will also be of benefit. The worthy ideals of shared care require shared information.

(ii) What are the local circumstances?

Patterns of care will differ from area to area and the precise functions and arrangements of the register will need to reflect these local arrangements. The register will need to be "owned" by the various professionals in the locality.

(iii) Which health care professionals need to be involved?

General practitioners increasingly work in extended health care teams. Practice nurses are becoming more involved in the management of patients with chronic diseases. In our diabetic audit practice nurses played a major part in designing the project and in collecting the data. Without their involvement and support we would not have achieved such a comprehensive audit of our diabetic patients. It is vital that all the various health care workers involved in provision of a service are also involved and understand the functions of the register.

(iv) What information to collect and how will it be recorded?

The quantity of information required by the register should be kept to an essential minimum and be considered realistically achievable by the practice. Practice circumstances will vary and a register designed to allow different levels of data entry may encourage involvement. This is a feature of the FHS Computer Unit Diabetes Care Management System—Dialog[10].

The method of recording needs to be considered and duplication of data entry avoided if at all possible. Compatibility with current general practice computing systems will be necessary to avoid duplication.

(v) What information can be fed back to the practice?

Data flow must be two way and information fed back to the practice must be concise and relevant to the needs of that practice. Well designed standard reports may be sufficient but there should be scope to provide more specific information on request.

(vi) What educational support will be provided?

Quality feedback to the practices will result in educational needs being highlighted. These are unlikely to be unique to each practice. Appropriate educational support needs to be considered by those responsible for running the register.

(vii) What resource provisions are available?

Resource provision needs to be considered in two principle areas. First, will practices receive any direct reimbursement for their work in providing information to the register? Second, as and when deficits in service provision are highlighted, will any resources be available to meet these deficits?

(viii)   Who will have access to the data?

Issues of confidentiality need to be carefully addressed from the outset. Practices are likely to have concerns surrounding patient confidentiality and also the confidentiality of their own practice data. Fears of practice performance being policed via the register will need to be convincingly dispelled.

Conclusion

The successful operation of an accurate, comprehensive, population based register conjures up the image of computers manned by technocrats with obsessional tendencies. These skills are undoubtedly required but our experience has been that the people directly involved in the patients care need to be motivated and involved in the project if the necessary data is to be collected in the first place.

This may seem common sense but the Clinical Standards Advisory Group report on Standards of Clinical Care for People with Diabetes, in stating the obvious desirability of diabetes registers, went on to say[8]:

> *3.24   "Nowhere had a comprehensive population based register been established, there being no incentive to supply the necessary details by general practitioners not engaged in structured diabetes care."*

GP Located Registers

KEY POINTS:

Clearly defined practice population

Information from a single source

GP able to identify patients

GP able to provide valid data

References

1   Ward, J. D., MacKinnon, M., "Purchasing for quality: the provider's view" *Diabetes care, Quality in Health Care* 1 (1992), 260–5

2   Mant, D., Tulloch, A., "Completeness of chronic disease registration in general practice." *British Medical Journal* 294 (1987), 223–4

3   Donaldson, L., "Registering a need." *British Medical Journal* 305 (1992), 597–8

4   Howitt, A. J., Cheales, N. A., "Diabetes registers: a grassroots approach." *British Medical Journal* 307 (1993), 1046–1048

5   *Report of the Clinical Guidelines Working Group, Royal College of General Practitioners.* "The development and implementation of clinical guidelines." (1995)

6   Effective Health Care. "Implementing clinical practice guidelines." *Institute for Health, University of Leeds* (1994)

7   Thomson, R., Lavender, M., Madhok, R., "How to ensure that guidelines are effective." *British Medical Journal* 311 (1995), 237–42

8   *Report of a CSAG Committee.* Second Government Response. "Standards of clinical care for people with diabetes." (HMSO, 1994)

9   *The Diabetes Control and Complications Trial Research Group.* "The Effect Of Intensive Treatment Of Diabetes On The Development And Progression Of Long-Term Complications In Insulin-Dependent Diabetes Mellitus." *New England Journal of Medicine* 329(14) (1993), 977–986

10 Vaughan, N. J. A., "DIALOG—the solution to creating a district diabetes register?" *Practical Diabetes International* Vol12 No3 (1995), 114–116

4.2 Personal Experience with a District Diabetes Register System — Dialog Linked to the FHSA Database for Co-Ordinating Diabetes Care:
Design and Implementation

Dr N J A Vaughan, Consultant Diabetologist, Royal Sussex County
Hospital, Brighton

Introduction

The creation of district diabetes registers is seen as one of the high priorities for diabetes care which is enshrined in the St Vincent Declaration targets[1]; 'to establish monitoring and control systems using state of the art information technology for quality assurance of diabetes health care provision'. Within the recent recommendations of the Clinical Standards Advisory Group for diabetes[2], as well as in the joint Department of Health / British Diabetic Association St Vincent Task Force (DH/BDA SVTF) report this need is further reinforced. Population based information on the process and outcomes of care are an essential aspect of the continuing audit of diabetes services[3] for needs assessment and will be fundamental to securing resources for diabetes care through the commissioning process. In order to obtain population based data, it is particularly important that comprehensive data are obtained from primary as well as the secondary care sector. Already a number of excellent individual information systems exist in secondary care and a few general practices are also capable of collecting this type of information. However, only one or two systems have even approached the goal of collecting comprehensive population based data across a district[4,5]. This is perhaps an indication of the huge and difficult task that creating, and especially maintaining, a comprehensive register represents. High patient mobility, particularly in inner city areas, can make this an almost impossible task. If diabetes registers are to be a feature of every diabetes service then a simple inexpensive solution for developing a register must be found.

The introduction of chronic disease management clinics by the majority of general practices to provide diabetes care has necessitated the development of practice diabetes registers and begins to simplify the task of creating district diabetes registers. Clinical information from the process of diabetes annual review is being routinely recorded in the clinical record but this activity needs to be coordinated in a manner that ensures it is not only conducted to an agreed formula or dataset but that a mechanism is in place centrally to aggregate this data. Individual enthusiasts have shown that this is possible on a limited scale but a widely applicable approach has not emerged, although the adoption now of a standard UK diabetes dataset[6-9] is an important first step. The development of DIALOG[10-12], the Family Health Services Computer unit (FHSCU) system for diabetes care management, potentially offers a solution to this problem, both for prompting the diabetes annual review process and accumulating clinical information on a district diabetes register across both sectors of care.

In the United Kingdom there already exists a population register that is maintained by the national Office for Population Censuses and Surveys (based at Stockport in the Midlands). This is linked to administrative registers held and maintained in every health authority (HA) area by the Family Health Services Authority (FHSA). There are 90 FHSAs in England alone varying in population size from 300,000 to in excess of 1 million. The principle purpose of these registers is for managing primary care services. These local FHSA registers are regularly updated, a process involving a substantial amount of work. In an average district of 750,000 population there may be 12,000 amendments to the register per *week*. This register has formed the basis for the breast and cervical screening programmes and has obvious potential for population health care.

It was therefore of great potential significance that in 1992 stakeholders representing the FHSA decided to commission a Diabetes Care Management System, now called DIALOG. This system is linked realtime with the FHSA population register, greatly simplifying the burden of maintaining any register, and is able to act as an interface between the primary and secondary care diabetes information systems (Figure 1).

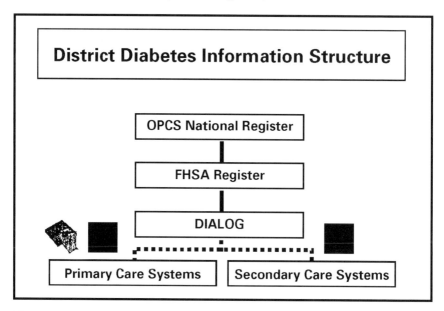

Figure 1

However, although DIALOG may have the desired functionality, it is the organisation within which it operates that will determine its success. This poses a dilemma for some clinicians. DIALOG has been designed by the Family Health Services Computer Unit (FHSCU) and is intended to work in close proximity to the main FHSA register, although a stand-alone option is also available. The uneasy relationship over the past few years between primary care and the FHSAs in some parts of the country immediately arouses suspicion and disquiet amongst clinicians at the idea of the FHSA holding clinical data, although in fact they already hold a significant amount of such data in other clinical areas. Any implementation of DIALOG must take account of this and create a structure to absolutely ensure the security* of the information and to assure the clinicians (and patients) that it will only be used and interpreted in an agreed manner. This is probably a role of the local diabetes services advisory group, or nominated subgroup, and will be critical to the register's acceptance. It also means that clinicians, public health and the FHSA, or new health authorities, must work amicably together in the common interest of providing quality diabetes care.

This paper goes on to describe the way that DIALOG has been successfully implemented in the Brighton, Hove & Lewes localities of East Sussex Health Authority, a population of 300,000 served by one District General Hospital (Brighton Healthcare Trust) with two consultant diabetologists and having 64 general practices, ranging from many single-handed general practitioners to large medical centres. This process has been described elsewhere in detail[12].

The Design and Development of the Dialog System

DIALOG is a computer software application that has been written by the FHSCU, an agency at arms length from the Department of Health. These groups have previously developed the National Cervical and Breast Screening Programmes. In 1992 a steering committee was established including representation from the British Diabetic Association, general practitioners, members of FHSAs, public health, health promotion with an observer from the Department of Health. From this group emerged the concept of a system that would fulfil the functions of a diabetes register, that would prompt the essential process of the diabetes annual review for individual patients and could also collect and aggregate clinical information. After a great deal of discussion and wide consultation, by the summer of 1993, a design specification for the system had been produced. This then underwent the necessary development phase of logical design followed by detailed review and modification by the steering group. The process was managed through 'PRINCE' project management methodology. Subsequent user acceptance and evaluation of the product resulted in a few further

The Department of Health has issued guidance on security of data and more recently issued new guidance on confidentiality in March 1996

minor modifications, and finally several centres around the country undertook pilot implementation of the prototype system, each centre using the application in a slightly different way in order to test its robustness and flexibility. This process was completed in November 1994 and DIALOG has been made generally available.

The primary aim of the DIALOG project was to define and develop a system to assist in the care of people with diabetes, through the organisation of a recall structure specifically for the diabetes annual review examination. Thus, the objectives were to develop software to facilitate this process. The following functions (figure 2) were specified as essential:

1   Maintainance of a register of individuals with diabetes with clinical information stored against this register.

2   Recall of patients with diabetes for Annual review with appropriate notifications.

3   Summarised individual clinical diabetes data which can be transferred when a patient changes diabetes registers. This also provides a mechanism to ensure that the individual patient remains known to the care provider.

4   Recording of clinical information ascertained from the patient's annual reviews. This is intended to ensure patients receive a consistent level of care and facilitates monitoring of outcome.

5   Provision of a system based on the minimal level of care as outlined both in the British Diabetic Associations 'Patient's Charter' (What care to expect) and the St Vincent Declaration.

- **Maintainable register of patients with diabetes and clinicians**
- **Recall facility for Diabetes Annual Reviews**
- **Storage of clinical data from Diabetes Annual Reviews**
- **Manual or disk (ASCII format) input information**
- **National standard clinical dataset and codes used throughout**
- **Detailed statistical reporting**

Figure 2:   Summary of the functions of Dialog

It was also recognised that DIALOG might be required to be able to run in 2 modes:

Integrated mode—linked physically to the FHSA registration database to enable realtime download of demographic data. The items brought across being:–

Patient's surname

Patient's forenames

Patient's sex

Patient's date of birth

Patient's address

Patient's GP

GP's name

GP's address

Stand-alone mode where the system is held on a seperate machine with no electronic linkage to the main FHSA system and thus must maintain its own registration database.

The design specification embraces these features and can be divided into a number of functional areas which are described.

The Functional Areas of the Dialog System

1 Diabetes District Register

DIALOG is a maintainable register of patients with diabetes and clinicians involved with each patients diabetes care. By far the most important feature of DIALOG is it's ability to create a diabetes register through its utilisation of the FHSA register's demographic information. In the first instance details of patients under a clinician's care must be passed to the system, either as a physical list or as electronic data on a flat file ASCII diskette.

DIALOG assumes the fundamental role of requiring the identification on the register of the lead clinician—the person who is going to take prime responsibility for performing the diabetes annual review each year. This may be the general practitioner, or the diabetes specialist, if the patient is seen regularly in hospital or at the local diabetes centre. It can also deal with the situation where the lead clinician works at several sites. If the lead clinician is someone other than the patient's general practitioner, the GP is recorded as the secondary clinician. The lead clinician, however, is not fixed permanently, it can be changed if the patient's care is transferred from one sector to the other. The pattern of use for this function may vary from district to district, especially where formal shared care schemes may already be in operation. The system is deliberately very flexible, being very easily configured to meet local need. This function does however ensure that an identified clinician is always responsible for the annual review.

When initially creating the register, the download of data to DIALOG must include the patients surname, forename and date of birth, and can also include: hospital identifier, ethnic origin (national code), diabetes status, year of diagnosis, lead clinicians details (national code), location of treatment (code), secondary clinician details (national code) and date of annual review. DIALOG can also provide the NHS number (the only unique patient identifier) to secondary care providers. Considerable care has been exercised throughout the design of DIALOG to use national codes wherever these exist in order to facilitate the possible transfer of data between systems without potential ambiguity.

2   Diabetes Annual Review Process

DIALOG provides a recall facility for the process of the diabetes annual review for an individual patient. This is a key feature of the provision of any diabetes care and the system will prompt the annual review each year. When the system is first set up it must be provided with the date the lead clinician would like to undertake the annual review process. This can be set in various ways; it may just follow on from the previous years annual review, or it can relate to a particular process of the annual review, eg fundal examination. If a date is not specified the system will default to the patient's birthday.

- **Prior Notification Lists** The system first issues a prior notification list (PNL). The PNL is a list of those patients whose diabetes annual reviews are due within a specified period. Both the frequency of the issue of PNLs and the interval before the annual review is due can be configured by the users to suit their local requirements. The PNL gives details of the lead clinician, minimum patient identification data (ie NHS number, hospital identifier, name, address, date of birth, and the general Practitioner's name and address, the date of expected annual review and an area for amendments). The PNL alerts the lead clinician that the annual review is due.

- **Clinical Data Sheets** At the same time as the prior notification list is issued a clinical data sheet is generated to record data gathered at the annual review. It is anticipated that the clinical information requested may not necessarily all be gathered at the same time and it is intended that any of the procedures or tests performed within the last 12 months should be recorded. Return of the completed clinical data sheets will cancel any further reminders until the next annual review is due. The clinical data sheets can be issued for the three levels of data entry specified in the UK diabetes standard dataset[9]. These are automatically produced by the system and have been carefully constructed to conform with the data entry screens to facilitate manual input.

In subsequent years the clinical data sheets that accompany the prior notification lists will also record the previous year's entries so that only items that have changed will require re-entry. This attempts to keep the paper work to a minimum and further developments of the system will address ways in which duplication of record making can be minimised.

If existing information systems can deliver data in the electronic ASCII format specified with the UK dataset[9] this is accepted by DIALOG and will greatly assist the process of data transfer. Discussions are underway with primary care software systems suppliers to develop means of facilitating the electronic transfer of data from general practice, particularly where local networking via 'GP Links' may be in use. Any information held on DIALOG can be transferred with a patient's details when he moves from one FHSA area to another.

- **Storage of clinical data from annual reviews** The database and clinical data sheets issued by DIALOG employ the UK diabetes dataset that has been developed and piloted by the joint British Diabetic Association and Research Unit of the Royal College of Physicians Audit Working party[6-9]. It is also compatible with the European dataset—DIABCARE as well as supporting Read Codes. However, this dataset is large and it was felt to be too formidable to be realistically employed at the outset, especially where Primary care is concerned. Thus, the hierarchical data structure, with three levels of increasing complexity, has been adopted to enable phased introduction of data collection[8]. Each level of data structure has been incorporated into DIALOG as a specific suite of screens, so that one can predetermine for an individual patient or practice, the amount of data collection required. On entering the DIALOG system one can select the desired level of data entry, ie the minimum dataset (level 1), the intermediate dataset (levels 1 and 2) or the full dataset (levels 1, 2 and 3). The first level (Appendix 1) amounts to 32 data items, 10 of which are demographic information already contained in the FHSA register. This still gives very useful process and outcome data for diabetes care. The second level contains a further 20 items, and the full dataset has 99 fields, although once recorded many items will not change year on year (and a substantial number of fields represent alternative measures, ie HbA1, HbA1c and fructosamine represent three fields, although it is likely that only one of these will be recorded). It is intended that this structure will enable an incremental approach, perhaps over several years, to data accumulation eventually aiming to gather the full dataset across the entire population. However, within DIALOG there is nothing to prevent one collecting one's own subset of data if there are specific items required that did not conform to the provided structure.

- **Recall letters** There is also an option for the system to automatically issue recall letters to patients if this is desired. This function may be of particular benefit to general practices. The letter indicates to the patient that their annual review is due shortly and that they should make contact with their doctor to have this done, unless arrangements have been made to do this already. DIALOG can issue a series of reminder letters both to the lead clinician, if a clinical data sheet has not been returned, and a final notification to the general practitioner, whoever is responsible for performing their annual review, if the patient has failed to attend. The timing of the letters for recall and the reminders can be configured to suit local requirements although the default timings of this whole process of attempted recall lasts 4-6 months. If the patient does not respond, no further action is taken until the next annual review is due and then the whole process will start again. Prior notification for individual patients, in whom perhaps annual review may be inappropriate, can be inactivated but such patients will remain on the register.

3   Statistical Reporting and Management Information

DIALOG can deliver detailed statistical reports easily and regularly for any individual lead clinician or groups of patients. The reports are based on those specified by the UK Audit Working Party[6,7]. Each lead clinician should receive grouped data analysis for his patients and optionally, aggregated reports for both Primary and Secondary care can be produced for information and comparison. Oracle, through its SQL (standard query language) will also permit more specific customised reporting if required. It should be stressed that, at least at this stage in the development of DIALOG, it is not intended that general practitioners can directly access information held about a particular patient. It is assumed that such information would be held locally on clinical management systems.

DIALOG will be able to deliver aggregated anonymised information in an electronic form that can be analysed centrally for comparison with other areas (as undertaken in the joint British Diabetic Association and Research Unit of the Royal College of Physicians audit feasibility study[6,7]) and also in a format that is compatible with the DIABCARE Quality Network (Q-Net)[13]. This facility is obviously important in the event that a National Register/Database is ever established.

4   Maintenance of Other Registers

At the discretion of the system managers (clinicians) concerned DIALOG can provide administrative and Registration data to other clinicians or diabetes Registers when a patient changes clinician/FHSA. Similarly, clinical data can be transferred to other systems, if this is felt to be appropriate, when patients move. Whenever a patient is deducted (removed) from the register, either because he has moved or died the lead clinician is notified. These notifications can be sent at specifiable intervals, generally monthly. This is particularly valuable for secondary diabetes care registers, as generally this information is difficult to obtain, delayed or never appears.

5   Administration Screens

A series of administrative screens enables parameters of the system to be configured to local requirements. These also serve to control printer functions, enrol new users, backup and retrieval.

6   Creation and Maintenance of the Diabetes Care Recall Registers

This part of the system enables creation of the database, both manually and from disk, input of new and amended patient registration details, as well as deletion of patient details. A Clinicians register can also be created with site codes.

System Technical Requirements

DIALOG has been written using Oracle[a] with a relational database. A relational database allows data to be accessed more easily and there is a multitude of compatible report writing packages available. Oracle[a] is a market leader in fourth generation languages and relational database management systems and is now becoming a standard software application within the health service. It runs under a Unix operating system and will run on any medium sized personal computer (minimum specification 486DX 50MHz processor, 500Mb hard disk, 16Mb RAM) either physically linked to the FHSA system or standing alone. Where linked to the FHSA computer, a Ethernet Card and communication software (MSM, MSMAPI and NSMNET) will also be required. A form of backup media will be necessary to perform routine backups of the system such as a tapestreamer that can hold at least 200Mb of data.

Data Security and Confidentiality

The storage of clinical data is an extremely sensitive issue wherever it is held and great care has been taken with security of the system to ensure data confidentiality, although ultimately this must be the responsibility of the system managers. Where DIALOG is linked to the FHSA computer it is invisible to any user of the main FHSA register and cannot be accessed through this system. No record appears upon the FHSA system indicating that an individual has diabetes. Password access to DIALOG is required and if DIALOG is installed on a seperate personal computer linked electronically to the main FHSA system, there is also has the advantage that this machine can simply be turned off when not in use. This offers much greater control over who uses the system. For the future, encryption is being examined as an additional means of securing the data. It is probably also appropriate that a local 'Data Ownership Committee' with representation of all interested parties is established to control* access, use and interpretation of such data.

* In line with new DH guidance on confidentiality this committee could only agree guidelines for access.

Cost

A description of the system would not be complete without an indication of the likely cost of the system.. These are not finalised but approximations would suggest the following: capital expenditure for setting up costs will include hardware, which is unlikely to exceed £3000 for the PC and a good laser printer will be required although this may already be available. Then there are the licenses for Oracle, the communication software and the Unix operating system, this will depend upon the anticipated number of users but is likely to be between £3000 and £6000. (For the stand alone version deduct £1000 for the communication software licenses. Subsequent revenue costs for the system support are likely to about £3000 per annum.

A Model for Implementation of Dialog

Initially two sites, Brighton and Brent and Harrow agreed to pilot the FHSA linked version. Both centres are now successfully running the system for both primary and secondary care[11]. A number of technical problems were identified during the piloting phase that have subsequently been addressed through the DIALOG user group and the Family Health Services Computer Unit have implemented appropriate corrective action. There has also been strong interest from districts all over the UK with numerous demonstrations by the active sites of this solution to the creation of a district diabetes register. Already, several other centres have adopted the system and are in the process of implementation.

Process of Implementation

1   Initial Consultation and Planning

It became apparent fairly early on in the development of DIALOG that, in piloting the system, testing the software would be the easiest part. Implementing it within the district organisation of a diabetes service would be the crucial test of its acceptability and longer term viability. Initial approaches were therefore made in writing to the East Sussex FHSA and the Public Health Department of East Sussex Health Authority, about 12 months before the system was installed. This engendered sufficient interest to make it worthwhile meeting informally to discuss the project further.

Informal discussions The first meeting included a consultant diabetologist, the Director of Business Services for the FHSA and a consultant from Public Health. The concept of DIALOG was outlined. Particular emphasis was placed upon it's ability to gather population based data and the way this would be consistent with the district philosophy for diabetes care. As all parties expressed enthusiasm for trying to proceed, it was felt that the next step would be to take a proposal to a specially convened meeting of the District Diabetes Advisory Group. A number of other relevant individuals were also invited to this meeting.

Local Diabetes Services Advisory Group This group, at that time, included representatives from the hospital Diabetes Centre, Local Medical Committee (LMC) of general practitioners, Department of Public Health, Director and Information Manager of FHSA, FHSA Nurse Adviser, and one of the Locality Commissioners. A proposal was outlined for implementing DIALOG, to be physically sited at the FHSA headquarters in order to take advantage of electronic linkage with the FHSA computer. It was clear that there were going to be funding implications both for the likely hardware and software requirements and as a result of the proposed post of a diabetes district register Manager. This latter item was seen as an essential determinant of the project's success. A steering group was established to undertake further detailed planning and to report back to the Local Diabetes Services Advisory Group.

Steering Group This comprised a consultant diabetologist, a senior registrar in Public Health, the Director of Business Services for the FHSA, the diabetes register manager, a nurse adviser and a general practitioner from the Local Medical Committee. Meetings were on a monthly basis to plan and monitor the implementation of DIALOG. The senior registrar in Public Health, who was elected chairman of this group, also undertook to evaluate the process of implementation and to validate the data that was collected.

Role of Diabetes Register Manager It was clear that in order to successfully operate the register an identifiable individual must be responsible for administering DIALOG. This person should be answerable to the Local Diabetes Services Advisory Group or their nominated representatives. It was felt that it would be an advantage for the Diabetes Register Manager to have previous experience of how the FHSA register operates and in particular how the screening section of the FHSA (Cervical and Breast screening programmes) functions. This also simplifies the issue of data entry which is undertaken both by the diabetes register manager and also specified individuals in the Screening Department at the FHSA. The first task would be to become familiar with the DIALOG software and then load a copy of the hospital register, matching patients with the main register. At the same time, it would be necessary to arrange visits to all general practices explain the system. Personal contact with clinicians in primary and secondary care is be an important aspect of the job. It was envisaged that initial training would be required for general practitioners and practice nurses to familiarise them with DIALOG's outputs and in particular with completing the clinical data sheets. Where practices have not already established a diabetes register the diabetes register manager could offer administrative help in compiling this.

Funding A number of sources of funding were explored including both Regional and Local Audit Committees, Regional Information Strategy Group and Primary Care Development Fund. In the end, full funding was obtained from the Regional Information Strategy Group for the first year and ongoing funding has now been secured from the Locality Commissioners. An approximate annual salary cost of the District Register Manager is £15,000.

Register Compilation

Populating the register is perhaps the most difficult aspect of the entire project. There is simply no easy way of doing this; the most difficult group to pick up reliably being those patients with non-insulin dependent diabetes managed with diet alone. It was decided that this should be tackled in several ways including a direct approach to patients inviting them to self-register.

1 Diabetes Centre Register Download

A hospital based register of patients has been in existence for 6-7 years. This was held as part of a clinic based computerised information management system, 'Diabeta II' (a version of the computer system 'Diabeta I' developed at St Thomas's Hospital and extensively modified in conjunction with the audit feasibility study conducted by the joint working group of the British Diabetic Association and Research Unit of the Royal College of Physicians). This system gathers clinical data 'live' at every clinic attendance, both interactively and through paper proformas. In addition, a computerised District Retinopathy Screening Programme had over a similar period identified a further substantial group of patients. The two registers together amounted to about 4,500 patients, approximately three–quarters of the predicted diabetic population (based on a prevalence of 2%). Both registers are linked to the Hospital Patient Administration System. The hospital diabetes register was downloaded in a flat file format on diskette and loaded into DIALOG, simultaneously matching patients with the FHSA database. Of 2,800 registrations, 2042 were current, 300 were from adjacent districts, 100 were not readily identifiable (inconsistencies in demographic information), and had to be individually checked. The remainder were dead or had moved from the FHSA area and had not been archived. Correct matching enabled delivery of the NHS number into a further file to be read back into the hospital register. It was felt at this stage that to incorporate the information from the Retinopathy Screening register was inappropriate as many of these were not under the hospital's care. It is hoped that once all primary care patients have been identified, cross-checking can be used to discover any omissions.

Although technically this information could, under the Data Protection Act, be transferred between the two systems, it was felt that patients should be given the opportunity to opt out. Therefore, a letter explaining the system and indicating the intention of placing their names upon the register was sent to every patient. A declaration at the end of the letter, if signed and returned (freepost) would ensure their removal from the register. In fact only 8 out of 2042 patients decided they did not wish to be included, which confirmed the findings of a preliminary survey we had carried out in a specific practice (Personal communication Dr J Bennett, Mr A Prosser)

Subsequent operation of the DIALOG register has resulted in the issue of monthly updates to the hospital register, including deaths and removals to other FHSAs. This has proved invaluable and was previously virtually unobtainable. Receipt of Prior Notification Lists (PNLs)—a monthly list of those patients due for annual review, has enabled clinical data to be extracted electronically from the diabetes centre computerised database in file format and downloaded into the DIALOG system. We have found it most convenient to perform this task 4 weeks after the annual review was due. It has however enabled us to identify more readily patients not seen for over a year. Minor reorganisation of out-patient clinic lists for annual reviews has been necessary to try and recall these patients within a reasonable time period.

For all the diabetes centre patients, the data items contained within the full UK dataset have been transferred electronically to DIALOG. However, for a few individuals seen at a small diabetic clinic in another hospital, this operation has been undertaken manually. Completion of the full dataset proformas takes about 2 minutes, providing the hospital notes are already reasonably structured as far as diabetes related information is concerned.

2   General Practice Recruitment—Diabetes Roadshow

An individual approach to general practices was felt to be more likely to be successful in recruiting general practitioners to participate rather than a series of large meetings. This also gave an opportunity to discuss how DIALOG fitted into the overall district strategy for diabetes care. As well as providing time to allay fears about how the clinical data might be used. Naturally there was considerable anxiety that this was a way of monitoring activity that could be used punitively. It had been agreed from the outset with the Medical Director of the FHSA that this would in no way be linked to payments for Chronic Disease Management Clinics for diabetes, although participation in this scheme would guarantee such payments.

These meetings were held at lunchtimes at the practices, with refreshments, and approval was obtained for general practitioner's attendance to qualify for 1 hour Post-graduate Education Allowance (PGEA). All members of the primary health care team were encouraged to attend. Practices were selected in no particular order, although those involved with area networking via 'FHSA/GP Links' (a national programme of electronic linkage of general practice computer systems with the FHSA computer, developed by the FHSCU were seen early on because of the potential for using this electronic communication highway for transferring data.

A consultant diabetologist, the diabetes register manager and the senior registrar from the Department of Public Health attended every meeting. A relatively informal presentation using an overhead projector or portable peronal computer was delivered giving a brief pre-amble on the St Vincent Declaration activities[10], the Diabetes Control and Complications Trial[11], the British Diabetic Association's patients charter (what care to expect) and the Clinical Standards Advisory Group report on diabetes care[12] to outline the background to the project. A district philosophy of care was introduced, followed by detailed discussion of DIALOG's function and how it would involve their practice, in particular how clinical data held on the register would be handled through a 'Data Ownership Committee'. Finally, the role of the FHSA and the Commissioners was discussed. Once agreement had been obtained from the practice principals and nurses the Diabetes Register Manager arranged to revisit to obtain any existing diabetes register, or to provide help to identify the practice's diabetic patients. Several such practice registers have been identified as being very incomplete. Again each patient was notified of the intention to place them on the DIALOG register with an option to opt out.

Thereafter, prior notification lists would be sent monthly, along with the clinical information sheets. Anticipating general practitioners reluctance to undertake completion of a form containing the full UK diabetes dataset, the first level of this[8], provided by DIALOG, has been adopted for the first year. Personal experience suggests this takes about 30–45 seconds to complete. In subsequent years it is planned to gradually increase the number of data items requested. Several general practices are actively exploring how they can transfer the information electronically from their own systems.

At the time of writing well over three quarters of general practitioners have been approached and nobody has declined to participate. There has been no perceived difference in attitude towards DIALOG between fundholders and non-fundholders. The amount of clinical data held on the system is still limited as an annual cycle has not been completed yet. However, audit reports are already being generated as the feedback for this process of audit.

3   Self-Registration Scheme

There seemed no reason why patients should not be approached directly to encourage self-registration. This would overcome some of the potential difficulties of data protection and possibly also identify a proportion of those patients managed by dietary means alone. However, specific targetting seemed more appropriate than relying on patients finding leaflets at general practitioners' surgeries. The Local Pharmaceutical and Local Ophthalmic Committees were approached to see if they would be prepared to distribute a leaflet describing DIALOG and its aims to any diabetic patient they saw in the course of their professional activities. They readily agreed to this suggestion and so the text of a pamphlet was drawn up, which also included outlines of the BDA's patient charter. This was 'plain-Englished' and art work added by the Health Promotion department at the FHSA prior to professional printing. The pamphlets are given out by pharmacists with any prescriptions containing diabetes related medication or products (including reagent strips) and by optometrists to any patient identified as having diabetes. It is proposed to run this scheme for a year in the first instance and evaluate its effectiveness.

To encourage patients to register in this way a Freephone number was provided on the pamphlet enabling them to directly contact the diabetes register manager (or answerphone). Whenever a patient made contact an effort was made to confirm their details (especially their general practitioner) and their diabetes was confirmed with their practice. Although included in the register at this stage, no attempt was made to begin issuing reminders until the general practice concerned had agreed to participate in the register.

Maintenance of Register

Once the register has been created, there is the longer term problem of ensuring that all new patients are identified. In the District there are between 300–400 new patients with diabetes diagnosed per year. It was decided to tackle this in two ways. Firstly, a form would be sent to each practice monthly, with the prior notification lists, requesting details of any patients who had been discovered to have diabetes within the past month. Hopefully all established diabetics moving into the area would be picked up on the health screen offered by general practitioners when a new patient registers with a practice and notified in the same way. Secondly, a version of the self-registration leaflet would be given to each patient at diagnosis as part of the information pack they generally receive. Whenever new patients are seen at the diabetes centre the lead clinician designation is assumed by the consultant and DIALOG notified accordingly unless the general practitioner has specified otherwise. Similarly when patients are discharged DIALOG and the general practitioner are notified and the GP resumes the lead clinician role.

Data Ownership Committee

Wherever clinical data is held in a manner that enables a patient to be identified it is essential that this information is secure and can only be accessed by authorised individuals. Individual outcome data falling into the wrong hands, eg life insurers, could be very damaging for a patient. Even anonymised data concerning specific practices or hospital units could potentially be very sensitive if available to uninformed managers and used as performance indicators. Every effort has been made to ensure data confidentiality for the individual. For the purposes of analysis, aggregated clinical information from DIALOG must also be controlled not only in how it is used but also in how it is interpreted. A Data Ownership Committee was established to handle this. Essentially this is a sub-group of the Local Diabetes Services Advisory Group. The membership includes a consultant diabetologist, a general practitioner, representatives from each of the Local Medical Committee and the Local Medical Advisory Audit Group, a public health consultant, a FHSA representative, a nurse adviser and a patient. Terms of reference for this body were agreed and all aspects of data output are handled through this group.

FHSA Role

This is perhaps difficult to define as the FHSA have been closely involved with all aspects of the implemantation of DIALOG and there has been a general feeling of common purpose: namely the establishment of a structure for ensuring the delivery of high quality diabetes care in the district. Their professional expertise with the information technology aspects of managing DIALOG, or indeed any register, have been especially valuable. They are also familiar with many aspects of management of Primary Care that are unknown to those working in the secondary sector .

As far as access to the data held on DIALOG is concerned, besides password restriction, this is also controlled through a strict internal disciplinary code for individual records. Similar mechanisms are already in operation for other FHSA systems holding clinical information, e.g. cervical smears, breast screening, immunisation etc.. The availability of any clinical audit information held in the system can only be through the Data Ownership Committee*.

Public Health/Commissioner's Role

Public Health and commissioners alike have the responsibility of promoting, maintaining and improving the health of the population within their authority's defined geographic area. On this basis, the commissioners, were enthusiastic about the concept behind DIALOG and were involved in the project from the outset. Moreover, in consultation with Public Health, they decided to sponsor the ongoing development of the diabetes register and to assist with the evaluation of its formation. The idea of collecting outcome data is attractive to the Commissioning Agencies. It offers an opportunity to assess needs and to measure the effect of implementing change, especially in the context of their agenda to examine the balance of care between primary and secondary care. This may be seen as very important to the future resourcing of diabetes care.

Not surprisingly there is also a shared common purpose in ascertainment and validation of the clinical data held on the register. This can only be done on a sample basis but is an important aspect of establishing the register.

* HSG(96)18 now requires all health authorities to ensure that guidance for the NHS on the protection and use of patient information is fully implemented.

In the initial stages it is anticipated that the register will miss cases of diet controlled diabetes and some older people with non-insulin dependent diabetes but with time these 'missing patients' should form an ever diminishing proportion of the population with diabetes. On this basis, the diabetes register has been recognised as a venture where investment now, will reap medium (3–5 year) and long term (5–10 year) rewards.

Discussion

Outcome measurement is essential for the implementation of change for the purpose of health gain and realistically it is only in this way that continuing enhancement of the quality of care and the provision of optimal diabetes services can be achieved. That a District Diabetes Register is an essential pre-requisite for obtaining population based data is indisputable. Feedback of individual practice information with comparative aggregated data for both primary and secondary care can serve as important performance indicators for those practices interested in audit. We have found this is an approach that has been greeted locally with general enthusiasm, particularly the prospect of comparison with their peer practices. This benchmarking type of activity has been shown to be an important aid to quality improvement in many other spheres.

However, to undertake such data accumulation and analysis, information technology solutions are likely to be essential. Over the past decade or more, many diabetes information systems have been developed in secondary care. These have involved a large amount of intellectual as well as financial investment and it is relatively unlikely that any individual system is going to emerge as a national standard, nor are many of these system 'owners' likely to be ready to scrap their systems in favour of an 'preferred' alternative. Moreover, with several excellent user friendly commercial database packages available, hospital information technology departments are often keen to adopt this approach as an inexpensive but effective solution to developing a system, rather than purchasing a system specifically designed for another diabetes service with the inherent problems of making it fit to local needs. The adoption of the National diabetes dataset will to a large extent determine the configuration of a system, and as this becomes more widely used we are likely to see a convergence of the functionality of systems in secondary care without a need for a prescriptive approach to an IT system for diabetes. At the same time, once primary care system developers have sorted out immediate problems with meeting accreditation requirements it is probable that data collection and export systems for the chronic disease management clinics will become available.

DIALOG has tried to anticipate the likely development of diabetes information systems and is an inexpensive solution to population based data gathering that avoids conflict with current systems either in secondary or primary care. Functionally, it sits one step back from the clinical interface where data gathering is undertaken, the clinic management systems act as feeders to the DIALOG system. It attempts to integrate the existing District Information systems, ie primary and secondary care and the FHSA population register. Its purpose is to prompt the process of Annual Review without regard to which sector is caring for a patient and it aggregates the data at a central point within a District or Area.

Of course a particular attraction must be the use of the demographic data from the FHSA register. The task of creating and particularly *maintaining* a district diabetes register should not be underestimated. Population mobility and the scale of the numbers make this a substantial undertaking that, if it be conducted accurately, is likely to be very demanding upon scant resources. Furthermore, unnecessary duplication of the activity of continually updating the demographic data held on the register, when this is already being done nationally through the OPCS/FHSA systems is unlikely to be a hugely attractive way to use resources for diabetes.

It must never be forgotten that the effectiveness of an information system is only as good as the organisation within which it rests, and the quality of the data that is entered therein. Great attention has been paid to making DIALOG extremely flexible to ensure it can be adapted to local variations in practice, and yet still provide a district wide structure for diabetes care. Nevertheless, DIALOG will still need to reside within the district structure for diabetes and advisably, wherever it is physically located, it should be under the primary control of the Local Diabetes Services Advisory Group and closely supervised and 'owned' by the clinicians therein. This is especially important if the clinical data the system holds is to be valid and both used and interpreted in an appropriate manner.

To set up a district diabetes register on a routine and long-term basis across an entire district is a formidable undertaking that should not be underestimated. Patient mobility makes the task of maintaining a 'live' register very difficult. In this respect there is no doubt that DIALOG has significant advantages because it greatly facilitates the maintainance of an accurate register through its links to the national population database. The important issue, however, is whether siting the register somewhere other than in the district diabetes centre, especially at the FHSA, is sufficient of a disadvantage to discourage its implementation on a wider scale. Our experience would suggest this is not the case but it does require the careful establishment of a productive relationship between clinicians, FHSAs and Public Health Departments with mutual understanding of each others perspectives. It must be said also that the main impetus for setting up the system has come from the District Diabetes Centre, rather than the FHSA or Public Health, and that this has probably been an important factor in convincing primary care to participate. Implementation does, however, need a 'champion'. In this environment of cooperation, with adequate control of data collection and handling, the whereabouts of the system is probably immaterial. However, if pre-existing discomforts, particularly between the clinicians and FHSAs, cannot be settled or there is disinterest in diabetes care from the public health perspective then employing DIALOG may be difficult, although its concept and pedigree might be a persuading factor. Our situation may have been fortunate in that the working relationships were already reasonable.

In the main the introduction of the system has been well received by general practitioners and especially by practice nurses, who are the persons that in reality are probably going to undertake much of the work. The individual approach to practices is an important part of the implementation process. Visits of the kind outlined to 'sell' the system are time consuming but they have been very well received and probably represent time very well invested. The alternative approach of conducting large meetings often fails to attract the attention of the less interested practices, and there is the inherent danger that only one individual needs to express strong dissent to swing the whole gathering behind them. The success of the smaller meetings has often been apparent in that they have been quite difficult to conclude, follow-on discussions covering a wide range of aspects of diabetes care, particularly the way it is delivered in the practice and how they can make better use of the resources of the District diabetes centre. An important aspect of convincing general practitioners that the clinical data will not be used to their detriment has been the formation of a Data Ownership Group with a substantial representation from general practice.

- **collaboration between clinicians, FHSA and Commissioning agencies**
- **FHSA database link**
- **District Diabetes Manager**
- **use of Standard UK Diabetes dataset**
- **ownership of system by clinicians**
- **feedback to clinicians involved with diabetes care**
- **Data Ownership Committee**

Figure 3:   Key Success factors to the operation of DIALOG

The diabetes register manager is the key person in the administration of the system. Very importantly, this person represents an identifiable individual that practices can contact with questions and the register manager's attendance at all the roadshow meetings has enabled a relationship to be established with the practice nurses and general practitioners. The offer of subsequent help, where required, to develop practice registers has been perceived as helpful although seldom actually used.

The long term goal for distict registers must be for the whole exercise to be accomplished electronically with data fed from diabetes clinic management systems, whether in primary or secondary care. DIALOG with its connections to the FHSA system will also have access to the primary care communications network 'FHSA/GP Links' that is currently being implemented. This has important functional implications for the future. It will enable the whole process of data transfer to be transparent between primary care computer systems and the diabetes register . Utilisation of these national communication links will mean minimal additional cost for establishing direct linkage and also ensure reasonable security.

DIALOG has been shown to be effective in its role of creating a district diabetes register, of prompting the diabetes annual review process and collecting clinical information on the process and outcomes of diabetes care across a district population. Optimal implementation demands a considerable effort of organisation but once established it should continue to operate smoothly. Some reappraisal of the structure of care within the district has been necessary especially where the relationship between primary and secondary care is concerned but this has probably enabled progress to be made towards a more integrated approach. At its simplest DIALOG provides a protocol for diabetes care that can serve to improve the quality of care. An added benefit is the accumulation of aggregated clinical data that may demonstrate a need for increased resourcing of diabetes care.

Conclusion

DIALOG is unique in its ability to to interface with the national register structures for primary care, and it is likely to remain so for the foreseeable future. Integrating data from primary care with information already gathered by many hospital diabetes management systems is the key to population based data which is essential to measurable progress to the St Vincent Declaration objectives. DIALOG can fulfil these functions very readily, bringing together existing information systems. It creates a maintainable register of patients with diabetes, recording which clinician (general practitioner or specialist) is primarily responsible for performing the Diabetes Annual Review. It has a prompting and recall facility for the Diabetes Annual Reviews and can store the standard UK clinical diabetes dataset obtained from this process of Annual Review. Information can be fed to the system either manually, ie by paper proforma or electronically on a floppy diskette. Data export is also possible and it is capable of very detailed statistical reporting. If DIALOG were to be widely adopted it could form the basis upon which a national register of diabetes could be established very easily.

CLINICAL DATA SHEET

PNL Number   : 1
Lead Clinician   : (National ID code)
Clinic   :

Patient Details
NHS No   : XXXXXXXXX   Hospital No   :
Name   : Mr A. N. Other
Sex   : M   Date of Birth : 04-JUN-1921
Address   : 23, Street, Town,
Postcode   : ZZ1 1XX

Diabetes Status   : Diet treated Diabetes
Date of diagnosis   :
Next Annual review date : 01/95
Ethnic Origin   :
GP details   : Dr A. Doctor

Annual Review data
Annual Review date : [/ /]
- -

Management
Diabetic treatment   -   Diet : [   ]   - Tablet : [   ]   - Insulin : [   ]
- -

Measurements
Were measurements taken   : [   ]
Weight   (   )   : [   ]kg   Height (   )   : [   ] m
Blood Pressure - Systolic   (   )   : [   ] - Diastolic (   )   : [   ]
Visual Acuity   Right   (   )   : [   ] - Left   (   )   : [   ]
Hba1/HbA1c   (   )   : [   ]%
Fructosamine   (   )   : [   ]micromol/l
- -

Eyes
Were eyes examined   : [   ]
- -

Feet
Were feet examined   : [   ]
- -

Other diabetes related problems
Were other diabetes related problems examined   : [   ]
- -

Risk factors
Smoking   (   )   : [   ]
- -

Hospital or sick leave days
Admissions for   - Foot problems   : [   ]
                    - Hyperglycaemic emergencies   : [   ]
                    - Cardiac problems   : [   ]
                    - Other   : [   ]
- -

Education/patient activities
Dietitian attended   : [   ]   Chiropodist attended   : [   ]

Appendix 1: DIALOG entry level (minimal) clinical data sheet, ( ) denotes previous years entry and shaded area indicates information provided by FHSA register following initial set-up)

References

1   Krans, H. M. J., Porta, M., Keen, H., Staehr-Johansen, K., "Diabetes Care and Research in Europe: the St Vincent Declaration action programme" Implementation document—Second edition. (World Health Organisation Regional Office for Europe, 1995)

2   *Clinical Standards Advisory Group:* "Standards of Clinical Care for people with Diabetes." (HMSO,1994)

3   Vaughan, N. J. A., *for the Diabetes Audit Working Group of the Research Unit of the Royal College of Physicians and the British Diabetic Association.* "Measuring the Outcomes of Diabetes Care." *Diabetic Medicine* 11 (1994), 418–423

4   Bennett, I. J., Lambert, C., Hinds, G., Kirton, C., "Emerging Standards for Diabetes Care from a city-wide Primary Care Audit." *Diabetic Medicine* 11 (1994), 498–492

5   Hurwitz, B., Goodman, C., Yudkin, J., "Prompting the clinical care of non-insulin dependent (type II) diabetic patients in an inner city area: one model of community care." *British Medical Journal* 306 (1993), 624–630

6   Williams, D. R. R., Home, P. D., and members *of a Working Group of the Research Unit of the Royal College of Physicians and the British Diabetic Association.* "A proposal for continuing audit of Diabetes Services." *Diabetic Medicine* 9 (1992), 759–764

7   Wilson, A. E., Home, P. D., and members *of a Working Group of the Research Unit of the Royal College of Physicians and the British Diabetic Association.* "A dataset to allow exchange of information for monitoring continuing diabetes care." *Diabetic Medicine* 10 (1993), 378–390

8   Alexander, W., Bradshaw, C., Gasby, R., Home, P. D., Kopelman, P., McKinnnon, M., Redmond, S., Vaughan, N. J. A., "An approach to manageable datasets in diabetes care." *Diabetic Medicine* 11 (1994), 806–811

9   Vaughan, N. J. A., Home, P. D., *for the Diabetes Audit Working Group of the Research Unit of the Royal College of Physicians and the British Diabetic Association.* "The UK Diabetes Dataset—a Standard for Information Exchange." *Diabetic Medicine* 12 (1995)

10 Vaughan, N. J.A., "DIALOG—a solution for creating a Diabetes District Register?" *Practical Diabetes* 12 (1995), 114–116

11 Vaughan, N. J. A., Hopkinson, N., Chishty, V., *for the DIALOG Working Party of the FHS Computer Unit.* "DIALOG—co-ordination of the annual review process through a District Diabetes Register linked to the FHSA database." *Diabetic Medicine* 12 (1995)

12 Vaughan, N. J.A., Shaw, M., Boer, F., Billett, D., Martin, C., "Creation of a District Diabetes Register using the DIALOG system." *Diabetic Medicine* 12 (1995)

13 Piwernetz, K., Massi Benedetti, M., Krans, H. M., Johansen, K. S., *DIABCARE: Monitoring And Quality Development in Diabetes Care—Regional and National Implementation of The St Vincent Declaration.* Editorial. *Diabetic Nutritional Metabolism* 6 (1995) 307–309

4.3   Personal Experience with a Population Based Diabetes Register run by a District Diabetes Liaison Board and Located in a District Diabetes Centre

Dr Robert J Young, Consultant Physician & Honorary Senior Lecturer, Hope Hospital, Salford

Introduction

Salford is an urban population of 229,000 people. There is substantial deprivation with Jarman score greater than 30 in 50% of the population. Medical services are provided by 132 general practitioners operating from 67 practices; 30 practitioners are single handed; there are 8 general practice funds covering 35% of the population. There is a single district general hospital, Salford Royal Hospitals NHS Trust, which is one of the University Hospitals of Manchester Medical School. The tertiary referral Paediatric Centre for Manchester, Royal Manchester Children's Hospital at Pendlebury, is also located in the district and provides local as well as regional services.

In 1988 a group of general practitioners, physicians, diabetes specialist nurses and representatives of the health authority and FHSA got together to start planning an integrated diabetes care service. This was consciously modelled from the start on the quality cycle (plan, do, check, review). Between 1988 and 1992 the initial group grew into a full District Diabetes Liaison Board, comprising hospital consultants, diabetes specialist nurses, general practitioners, practice nurse representatives, hospital and community dieticians, hospital community chiropodists, FHSA representatives, DHA representatives, local optometric committee representatives, people with diabetes, paediatric services representatives, and contributions when required from ophthalmic nephrological, obstetric, vascular, surgical and orthopaedic colleagues. This group agreed district guidelines including a charter of care, structured preventative care protocols, and referral and discharge thresholds; they promoted the formation of a diabetes centre which was established ultimately in 1991; and they worked hard at practice team development along with education and training for all health care professionals involved in diabetes care.

An initial abortive attempt at introducing the final 'check' part of the cycle was tried during 1989 and 1990 but failed largely for organisational reasons. In 1992 with the aid of regional audit funding a District Diabetes Information System was developed, implemented successfully, and has since been running throughout the district involving all general practices and hospital clinics.

Diabetes Information System Principles

Performance Monitoring

As indicated above, the system was developed primarily to serve the quality performance monitoring requirements of the system of care. Knowing that effective primary and secondary preventative health care can markedly reduce the adverse bimedical outcomes for diabetes (St Vincent Declaration) we wished to ensure that our protocols for care which were based on this understanding were being applied consistently and comprehensively. As Grimshaw & Russell showed in 1993 (1) 'explicit guidelines do improve clinical practice in the context of rigorous evaluation'.

Outcomes

To monitor our performance we wished not only to record 'key process achievement rates' but to monitor intermediate and final outcomes. To this end we recognised that in order for the denominator to be valid, the system would have to be population based. We recognised, further, that in order to fulfil this aspiration, to avoid duplicate data entry, and to maintain the central principle of integrated care (ie all providers operating to the same standards), the system would have to be equally appropriate to primary and secondary care.

Confidentiality and Security

We took a proactive approach to confidentiality. From the outset general practitioners and their representative groups (the LMC and MAAG) and hospital based diabetes health care professionals felt secure with the idea that database should be held by the District Diabetes Liaison Board (not the FHSA or DHA) and that rules of access to individual patient records should be identical to those in respect of access to written patient records. Accordingly the system is fully password controlled, the passwords are encrypted, and only aggregated anonymised data is released after full consideration by the District Diabetes Liaison Board. On the individual patient perspective we took the view that people with diabetes should be involved in data recording from the start so that they would be fully aware of the date which was being held but they should have a clear opportunity to decline to be involved if they wished. This has not so far proved to be a concern*.

User benefits

Recognising that information systems are only as good as the quality of data which is input we wished to ensure that people would want to use the system because they found it actually helped everyday clinical practice. The fulcrum of the integrated care programme is the concept of annual structured preventative care for everybody with diabetes. The key processes which are known to have a substantial impact on the outcome of diabetes care are all embedded in this annual care review and of course they form part of the UK dataset (reference). With wide user involvement we therefore devised a data collection form which would prompt primary or secondary care providers to ensure that all aspects of the structured preventative care review were completed and which actually represented a configuration of the UK dataset. This includes a simple assessment of wellbeing (sickness impact, service satisfaction), review of risk behaviours (diet, exercise, smoking, alcohol), documentation of intermediate outcomes (weight, blood pressure, HbA1C, lipids), and early complication screening (blood pressure, proteinuria, foot examination, eye examination). We also sought to provide practical benefits such as printing of laboratory request forms, call and recall, chronic disease management payment returns for practices, letters of invitation to patients etc. To avoid duplication it was agreed that for patients whose care was located solely in general practice (40%) the annual review sheet would be completed there but that if the patient attended the Diabetes Centre, albeit usually only once a year for structured preventative care review, (60%) then that was where the responsibility would lie for collecting the information.

Feedback

In addition to ensuring that data collection was facilitated by support of care delivery, we were also concerned to provide all users with appropriate feedback. For people with diabetes this is still at the development phase but should be fully implemented by the end of 1995 (Figure 1). Practices receive individual patient performance reports and comparative reports (Figure 2,3). Specialist clinics likewise receive reports relating to key performance and outcome measures for their groups of patients (Figure 4). At the district level reports are produced facilitating the targeting of important service adjustments.

---

* DH guidance HSG(96)18 requires that patients are made fully aware of the broad purposes for which information about them may be used. This is essential to underpin all personal data use, including anonymised or aggregate data for management purposes.

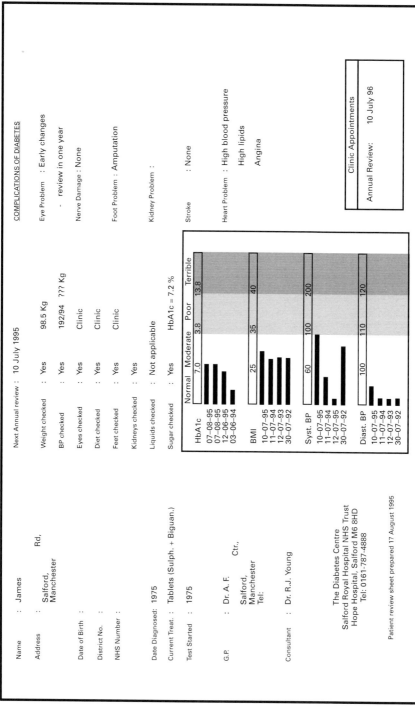

Figure 1

Performance data for GP: BUP14 (All entries)

Name	Hosp./NHS Nos.	Address	Diabetes	Eyes exam.	Feet exam.	Last HbA1c	Last lipids	Last BP	Last BMI
Dawn / DOB		Ave, Eccles, Manchester	Insulin By Pan Human	Yes 06-10-94	Yes 06-10-94	9.3	4.6/2.2	No BP measured	27.1
David / DOB		Road, Eccles, Manchester	Tablets Biguanides	Yes 11-05-95	Yes 11-05-95	8.2	6.1/4.7	135/90	30.8
Freda / DOB		Close, Eccles, Manchester	Diet	Yes 25-05-95	Yes 25-05-95	4.5	6.7/2.8	130/80	37.2
Bernard / DOB		Lane, Eccles, Manchester	Tablets Sulphonylures	Yes 22-06-95	Yes 22-06-95	5.2	5.0/2.0	158/90	27.7
David / DOB		Crescent, Eccles, Manchester		No	No	No HbA1c	No lipids measured	No BP measured	No Ht/Wt recorded
Kevin / DOB		Lodge, Street, Eccles	Diet	No	Yes 03-08-94	3.2	No lipids measured	110/75	No Ht/Wt recorded
Elizabeth / DOB		St PEEL GREEN Eccles	Insulin By Pan Human	Yes 28-06-94	Yes 28-06-94	8.9	4.7/1.8	130/80	26.7
Reginald / DOB		Road, Eccles, Manchester	Diet	Yes 08-06-95	Yes 08-06-95	No HbA1c	No lipids measured	130/80	76.9
Graham / DOB		Avenue, Eccles, Manchester	Tablets Biguanides	Yes 28-11-94	Yes 28-11-94	3.9	6.1/3.3	126/78	32.9
David / DOB		Road, Danton	Insulin By syringe Human	Yes 22-02-95	Yes 22-02-95	3.9	5.3/1.8	145/103	29.6
Andrew / DOB		Road, Eccles, Manchester	Tablets Sulph.+Bigun.	Yes 06-09-94	Yes 06-09-94	8.6	7.9/11.0	160/90	40.7
Elsie / DOB		Road, Eccles Manchester	Diet	Yes 24-08-94	Yes 24-08-94	5.9	No lipids measured	156/82	23.7
Maureen / DOB		Lodge, Street, Eccles	Diet	Yes 22-12-94	Yes 22-12-94	11.5	12.7/7.6	138/80	28.6
Lily / DOB		Road, Eccles	Tablets Sulphonylures	No	Yes 06-02-95	No HbA1c	No lipids measured	120/78	28.4

Figure 2

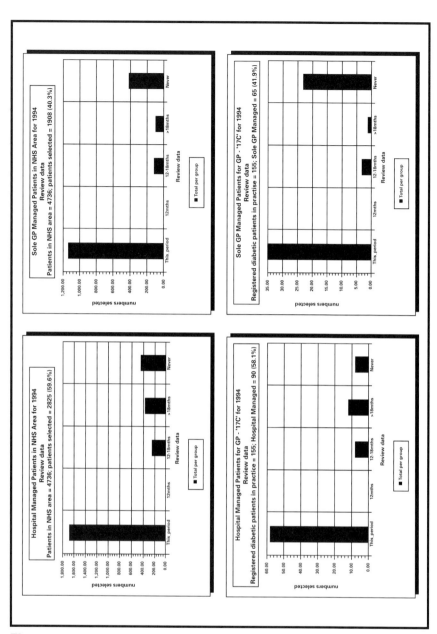

Figure 3

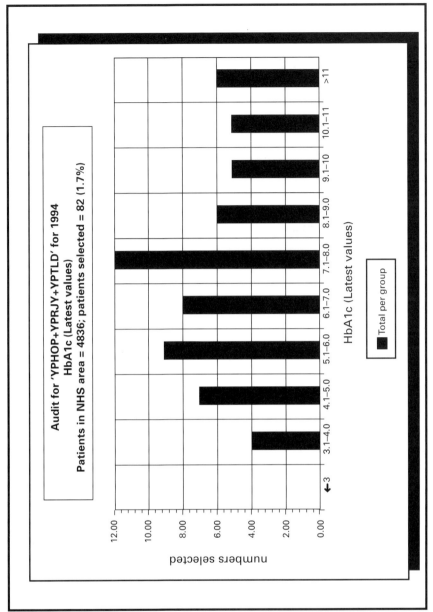

Figure 4

Practicality/Affordability

The final principle was to go for a 'low tech' solution which would be affordable, secure, appropriate to the wide diversity of provider locations, and, most importantly, endowed with adequate organisational support. It was our firm belief, on the basis of previous experience, that, without a committed system manager, implementation and maintenance in such a diverse organisational framework be totally impracticable. This belief has been fully supported by our experience and, we would suggest, has been the main determinant of success. The regional budget allocated was £15,000 per year. This has been supplemented, to a small extent, by other 'soft money' but has never exceeded £20,000 per year and the fully operational system now running operates within this budget. Given the huge direct and indirect costs attributable to diabetes this has seemed a reasonable amount to ask, if it will work. It is after all, less than the cost of one major amputation.

Operational Arrangements

Data is collected annually using the data collection form (Figure 5) at the time of the structured preventative care review. Distribution and collection arrangements for all the practices and specialist clinics have been worked out by the system manager. A letter of invitation to the review can be generated if desired and a laboratory request form is also produced automatically. At the time of the review a data collection sheet containing all previous information is available, and simply has to be updated. Standard clinical recording covers all the key processes (weight, blood pressure, foot examination, eye examination, metabolic control etc) as well as the listing of any new complications. Where the district general hospital laboratory has been used, biochemical data is automatically down loaded. The updated record is entered manually by the system manager or an assistant.

As indicated above final arrangements are being put in place for them ensuring that each patient receives a 'patient status report' from the system shortly after his or her structured preventative care review. Already in place are reporting systems to practices which provide lists of all their patients, individual patient performance in terms of the key processes, and aggregated comparative reports (own practice vs own practice patients attending Diabetes Centre vs all 'GP only' patients vs all Diabetes Centre patients (Figure 3). Lists of patients with no review recorded for more than 18 months whether the patient is supposed to be attending Diabetes Centre or practice have also proved popular and useful. Chronic disease management returns are routinely sent to practices for them to use if they wish. Individual clinics at the Diabetes Centre have found the 'service support' aspects of the system equally beneficial and information analysis in respect of the young person's clinic, the Diabetes renal clinic, the diabetes obstetric clinic and the general review clinic have all led to changes in practice already.

At the District Diabetes Liaison Board level the most obvious initial findings were the unexpectedly large prevalence of diabetes (2%), the high proportion of patients not receiving structured preventative care, and the low rate of retinal screening for GP only attenders. Consequent changes implemented between 1992 and 1994 are as follows: un-reviewed patients in general practice falling from 60.5% to 22.3% and in the Diabetes Centre from 44.5% to 16.2%; eye examination rising in general practice from 63.5% to 87.4%

SALFORD DISTRICT DIABETIC REGISTER

Surname:	District No.		Sex: M DoB:	Title: Mr.
Forenames: James			Ethnic Origin:	
Address: Rd,		GP: Dr. A. F.,		
Salford,		Health Ccr.,		
Manchester		Drive,		
		Salford.		
Postcode:	Hospital: HOP	Consultants: ROY	Date Diagnosed: 1975	

Current Diabetes Treatment

					Codes
Diet alone since (year) :					H = Human
Oral hypoglycaemics (year) : 1975	Sulphanyl : ☐	Biguanides : ☐	Bath : [+]		B = Beef
Insulin treatment (year) :	Syringe : ☐	By Pen : ☐	No. inj./days : ☐	Types : ☐	P = Pork

Complications

EYES	(Enter year)	FEET	(Enter year)	OTHER	
	Right Left		Right Left		Year
Cataract affecting vision	☐ ☐	Both foot pulses present	88 88	Proximal motor neuropathy	☐
Background retinopathy	☐ ☐	Sensory tuss		Other mononeuropathy	☐
Maculopathy	☐ ☐	Absent ankle jerk		Automonic neuropathy	☐
Pre-proliferative retinopathy	☐ ☐	Neuropathic pain		Impotence (req. treatment)	☐
Proliferative retinopathy	☐ ☐	Neuropathic ulcer		Soft tissue complications	☐
Retina not seen	☐ ☐	Claudication	93 93	Myocard. infarct	☐
Cataract extraction	☐ ☐	Tacheonic pain	90 ☐	Stroke	☐
Laser treatment	☐ ☐	Tacheonic ulcer	90 92		
Partially sighted	☐ ☐	Charcer foot			
Blind	☐ ☐	Amputation - Toe(s)	90 ☐		
		Amputation - Foot			
		Amputation - Knee	☐ ☐		

Values at last visit(s) — NOT TO BE COMPLETED BY DOCTOR

Date	HbA1c %	Glucose mmol/L	S-Creat. umol/L	Dual-Protein	U. Alb/Creat mg/mmol	Cholesterol mmol/L	HDL-chol mmol/L	Triglyc mmol/L	LDL-chol. mmol/L
07-08-95	7.2	22.4	113		3.22	6.5	1.06	5.1	
07-08-95	7.2								
07-08-95		22.4	113						
12-06-95	6.6								

Previous Review(s)

Date	Height metres	Weight kg	BMI	BP mm Hg	Hyperglyc. episode/yrs	Hypo.req assist/yr	Fundoscopy self	opt.	Oplith	Vis.ocuity R	L	Diet Disc	Refer	Feet Exam	Refer
11-07-94	1.88	93.60	26.5	154 /74	None	None	Y					Y	N	Y	N
12-07-93	1.88	94.50	26.7	142 /74	None	None						Y	N	N	Y
30-07-92	1.88	94.00	26.6	170 /80			Y					N	N	N	N

Clinical Review

Date	Height metres	Weight kg	BP mm Hg	Hyperglyc. episode/yr	Hypo.req assist/yr	Fundoscopy self	opt.	Oplith	Vis.ocuity R	L	Diet Disc	Refer	Feet Exam	Refer

Habits: Smoker None day	THERAPY: Lipid Lower.	Angina ☐	Snow on EYES: ☐	FEET: ☐	RENAL: ☐ Early ☐
Alcohol None units/wk	hypertensive	Card.Failure ☐	patient's		Moderate ☐
	Dial./T'plant	other (over) ☐	own form		Advanced ☐

Quality of Life

As a direct result of your diebetes, how many days within the past year :-
have you spent in hospital ? _____ days; have you not been able to work ? _____ days (or estimate if not working)
(not a lot) 1 2 3 4 5 (very much)
How much has diebetes been interfering with your life over the last year? : ☐ ☐ ☐ ☐ ☐
Are you happy with the diebetes care you have received over the last year? : ☐ ☐ ☐ ☐ ☐ (very happy)

Last Clinic	Annual Review	Return to sole GP to care	Medical Officer (Print)
10-07-95 15wks	10-07-95 * * NOW * *	YES/NO	

Please check and update ALL information. Shaded areas denote matching and revise data. (Amend HABLIS/THERAPY from prev. review)

Figure 5

and in the Diabetes Centre from 76.7% to 97.7%. Similar improvements are being achieved across a range of other process measures.

With regard to the St Vincent outcomes we are now in a position to produce overall district performance data which it will be possible, because of the uniform field definitions of the UK dataset, to compare with other districts. This is shown in the very preliminary retinopathy performance report (figure 6) which summarises primary prevention performance (glycaemic control), secondary prevention screening and treatment, and overall sight outcomes.

Salford District Diabetic Retinopathy Performance 1994

	GP	DC	District
Number of Patients	1923	2813	4736
Patients Reviewed	59.4%	59.4%	59.4%
HBA1c<7% NIDDM	80.1%	69.3%	73.4%
HBA1c<7% IDDM	43.5%	61.8%	61.3%
Eyes Screened	87.4%	97.7%	94.5%
New ST Retinopathy	15	64	79
ST Retinopathy ALLC	100%	100%	100%
Partially Sighted	2	2	4
Blind	0	0	0

Figure 6

Conclusion

We do not believe, on the basis of our own personal experience and discussions with many other districts, that there is a universal solution to the need for population based Diabetes Information Systems throughout the NHS. However a number of generic messages seem to have emerged from our experience thus far and these include:

- The UK dataset works; it is comprehensive and covers all the service support, quality assurance and reporting uses we have encountered to date.
- A system shared between primary and secondary care, and controlled by a district diabetes services group in the context of an integrated care system: is acceptable to users; can provide immediate tangible service support benefits; does not seem to violate any feelings of remote ownership; is easy to use; and it satisfies concerns about confidentiality.
- A system shared between primary and secondary care ensures a true population base, avoids data duplication, binds together an integrated diabetes care programme, facilitates communication and supports district service planning.
- Whereas sophisticated IT solutions will undoubtedly produce even more benefits, appreciable service support and very comprehensive reporting can be obtained with a simple PC based system which has a certain amount of intrinsic security.

- Tailoring a system which meets users needs and is maintainable to the local model of care is probably the biggest challenge for districts at the present time. A good manager, who works between care sectors, is essential.

References

1   Grimshaw, J. M., Russell, I. T., "The effect of clinical guidelines on medical practice: a systematic review of rigorous evaluations." *Lancet* 342 (1993), 1317–22

2   Vaughan, N. J. A., Home, P.D., *for the diabetes working group of the research unit of The Royal College of Physicians and the British Diabetic Association).* "The UK Diabetes Dataset; A standard for information exchange." *Diabetic Medicine* 12 (1995), 717–722

Legends

Figure 1   Draft version of patients status report
Figure 2   Individual patients key performance report
Figure 3   Comparative aggregated performance report for practices
Figure 4   HbA1C for a young persons clinic
Figure 5   Data collection form. The UK Dataset on one side of A4 as used by GP's and Diabetes Centre clinics in Salford
Figure 6   A district retinopathy performance report covering: primary prevention (HbA1C); secondary prevention (retinal screening and argon laser photocoagulation); and sight outcome

4.4   Personal Experience with the FHSA Population Register

Mike Cooke, Project and Business Manager, Family Health Service
Computer Unit, Exeter

Introduction

The Family Health Services Computer Unit (FHSCU) is an NHS organisation that reports directly into the Department of Health. Its main business is the development, support, maintenance of computer software for all 98 Family Health Service Authorities (FHSAs) in England and Wales. Because of our history with the Department of Health and FHSAs, I believe that the systems implemented within FHSAs are the only national systems in use within the NHS today.

The subject of my talk is the FHSA Population Register and what I propose to discuss now is the data that the FHSA Population Register contains; what it is used for; how the data is maintained; then to discuss the NHS strategy and standards and how that might help the discussion later on; and finally to consider some of the issues that FHSCU have come across in implementing Registers.

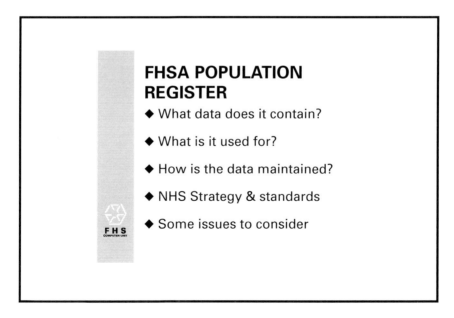

Figure 1

PATIENT DATA

One of the corner stones of the FHSA Population Register is its details of the administrative data about the local population (see attached handout). Some data items I would like to draw your attention to are the dates held about individual patients. These are date of birth, when they were registered with a general practitioner (GP) and when they were deducted i.e. when they left the FHSA area or died –there are a whole number of reasons for why patients would be deducted. Addresses, the address of a patient is linked to the post office address file and is fully postcoded; also preferred addresses are held if required. The address data is also hooked to grid references and various NHS organisation codes. The third item is the NHS number which is intended to be the unique identifier for individual patients and use of the new number will help in anonymising patient identification.

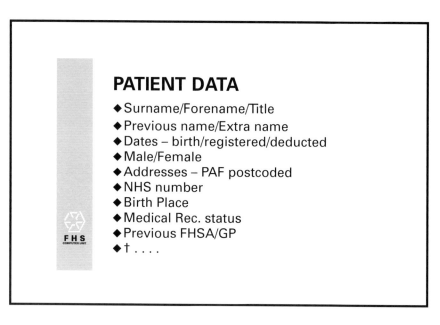

Figure 2

General Practitioner Data

Each patient is identified as having a specific GP for general medical services and the FHSA Register also contains a register of details about the GP (see handout for some of the key items for GPs held on the register).

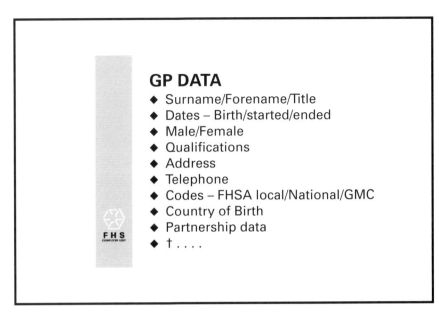

Figure 3

Uses of the FHSA Population Register

One of the main uses of the FHSA Population Register is that it records every patient registered with a GP for general medical services and is used to calculate the GP's capitation payment.

Medical Records Transfer is also another key function that the Population Register assists. Provision to the general public of prescription exemption certificates and monitoring of these.

There are currently two national screening systems that utilise the FHSA Population Register. These are the Cervical Screening programme and the Breast Screening programme. Both of these screening systems identified that the FHSA Population Register was the key national register for identifying women that fall into the various categories for screening.

What started with the two national screening systems has now turned into a major function of the FHSA Population Register, that is acting as a feeder system to other NHS registers.

USES?

◆ GP Capitation payments

◆ Medical Records Transfer

◆ Prescription Exemptions

◆ National Screening systems

◆ Feeder system to other NHS
registers

Figure 4

Feeder System to other NHS Registers

Because the FHSA has a statutory requirement to maintain the Population Register and a cross reference of patient to GP, it has been identified as one of the major sources of up to date information on patients and GPs. therefore, various links have been established to other FHSA Registers.

On this slide there are links between the various systems, two way links and one way links. The one way link is information flowing from the FHSA Register to the other NHS Register but not back to the FHSA, so data flows in one direction only. The 3 NHS organisations currently utilising the one way link are the UK Transplant Service and Support Agency (UKTSSA), who receive not only patient administrative details but also details about which organs they wish to donate. Dialog is the Diabetes Care Management System provided by FHSCU and can be run as stand alone or linked into the FHSA Register in order to get its patient administrative details. The third system is the NHS Administrative Register (NHSAR), currently there are 5 pilot sites within England and Wales that are populated from the FHSA Register in the first instance and in 2 of the pilots there is a one way link between the FHSA Register and the Administrative Register for patient admin details. The future plan, as I understand it, for the NHSAR is to initiate 2 way transfers of data between the FHSA and the NHSAR Registers.

Two way links are those where data is flowing in both directions between the various other NHS systems and the FHSA Population Register. One of the oldest of these is the hospital path lab links for Cervical Cytology data. This has been improved on over recent years. The NHS Central Register (NHSCR) at Southport has also been linked with all FHSAs for a number of years now, as have Breast Screening offices. The two national Child Health systems have been extensively piloted over the last 2 years and are now available nationally for all FHSAs to implement. Although the above systems have been around for a number of years, very few people seem to be aware of them because they operate without any problem. The latest links to go in are links to GP systems for the transfer of administrative patient data and registration transactions and more recently Items of Service for claims data. I believe this link to be a major success and is bringing major benefits to the NHS.

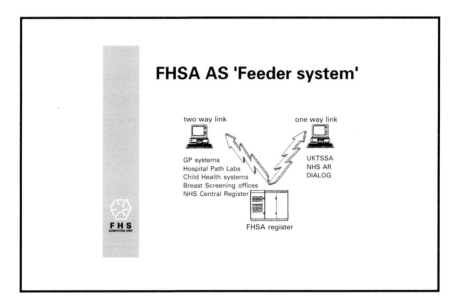

Figure 5

How Maintained

Before the advent of electronic links to other organisations within the NHS, the FHSA Register was maintained at the FHSA using VDUs to input and amend data. Some of the figures we used to publish were that across all FHSAs there were something like 5,000 on line terminals being used to input data that were based on paper forms from GPs, however, there are now 2,100 GP practices linked to FHSAs out of a total population of approximately 8,000 computerised practices and this figure will increase significantly over the next 18 months thereby reducing the need significantly for on line transactions from paper forms.

In building the electronic links many safeguards have been built into the systems that are now in place both for security and recoverability.

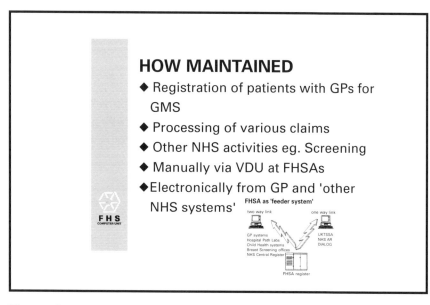

Figure 6

NHS IM&T Strategy/Vision & Principles

As part of the talk, I thought it would be worth mentioning the NHS IM&T Strategy as this gives a good lead to the NHS about how information systems should be used to work together for the benefit of the NHS. At FHSCU we are aware of the importance of having the strategy for the NHS and are constantly developing the systems we produce and maintain to ensure they adhere to the strategy and principles stated on this slide and the next.

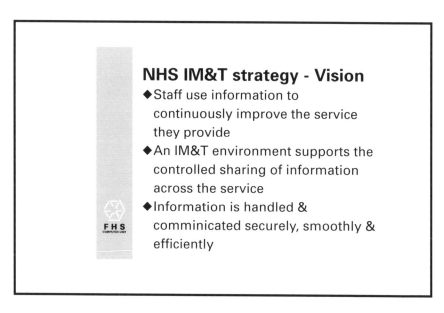

Figure 7

NHS IM&T strategy - Principles
◆Information will be person based
◆Systems should be intergrated
◆Information will be derived from operational systems
◆Information will be secure & confidential
◆Information will be shared across the NHS
◆Information should focus on Health

Figure 8

Issues

As part of this talk, I was asked to raise any issues that I felt appropriate based on experience that FHSCU have had so far. Some of these have been mentioned earlier but I will reiterate them here.

Reconciling Registers is no mean feat. What I mean by this is that in our experience of reconciling administrative data on patients between any other NHS Register is a big job, and something that should not be underestimated both in effort and elapsed time to do.

Once registers have been reconciled then keeping them in step is something that needs to be verified either by regular comparisons of data or via random checks. Currently there is a reconciliation exercise being undertaken by NHSCR to verify that the data they hold is in line with the data held at FHSAs. Considering the volume of transactions that flow between FHSAs and NHSCR and the number of years since the original take on and reconciliation was done the number of discrepancies has been very small, indicating that both systems are reliable and the data flows well defined.

ISSUES!

◆Reconciling Registers is no mean feat?

◆Once reconciled - keeping them in step?

◆Intergrated systems

◆Should there be a 'control' population register, locally based, that feeds & feeds from operational systems?

◆Data Protection - who can supply patients details to who?

Figure 9

Integrated Systems

There are a number of issues that I want to mention under this particular heading. The first is that any changes in one system need to be reflected in all of those that share that data. In order to share that data there needs to be adherence to NHS standards for data structures, in particular when we are looking at patient information, there is a common administrative dataset definition (CADS) that the NHS is encouraging. The second issue is that it is very difficult to get commercial suppliers of computer systems to change their systems unless they see any market advantage or benefit to them. Also the commercial system suppliers tend to have a long elapsed time in developing changes to systems and that once a system has been implemented they are not happy about implementing changes. Getting the changes agreed in the first place is a big exercise when you have a number of other systems that need to be in at the requirements analysis stage. The third issue is that by having a lot of linked systems, if a particular system allows wrong data to be entered, then the potential to spread that erroneous data throughout a number of other systems automatically is there. Therefore, there needs to be clear validation rules for data being entered onto the system and also, linked systems need to be accredited before being allowed to be hooked into the Network.

I believe there needs to be a master register that is controlled. If there isn't then the potential in linked systems that an update could end up going around in circles from one system to the other, each recognising it as a new change. Also for any audits or reconciliation a master register needs to be there such that it would have all the audit facilities in place to regularly check and validate its data. In the absence of anything else available within the NHS, I believe the FHSA Population Register is providing this facility at present.

Data Protection has been an issue for several years and will continue to be so in the future. There has been a lot of talk about confidentiality and not allowing patient details to be passed around within the NHS, however, I believe that the links that are in place with FHSA Population Registers are very secure and I am not aware of major confidentiality issues being raised over the 7 years that I have been working with this particular register. As long as we are all aware of the need for confidentiality and data protection and build security and audit checks into the systems that we produce, then the sharing of data across the NHS can only benefit the patient. Whilst I believe that organisations within the NHS need to keep their own data and registers locally, if these registers are not updated and maintained with changes related to patient administrative details and GP details, then that local database will soon start to degrade and will not benefit the patient in the long term.

As a post meeting note, I have been asked to discuss how the FHSA Population Register could be adapted to register patients with a variety of diseases.

As I discussed in the presentation, the FHSA Population Register has links to several other NHS registers for transmission of various types of data. Some of that data is clinical but the majority is to do with patient administrative details. One of the points that I was trying to make was that there is a need to maintain registers locally but that unless these registers administrative details are regularly updated, then the patient and GP details held on that register would become inaccurate and not reflect who the patient is currently registered with or where the patient lives etc. Hence my issue about having a master register that is the central repository for these administrative details and providing updates for other registers.

One of the problems with having a master register that provides updates to local registers, is that some of the local registers would be a small population size and therefore a small subset of a total FHSA Population Register for example. This means that within the FHSA Population Register there needs to be a flag or a series of flags, against a patient that identifies which other registers that patient is on. The FHSA Population Register software already has the mechanisms in place to be able to provide data to those other registers when there are changes to the administrative data related to that patient.

This is how the changes are sent to the UK Transplant Service and Support agency at Bristol. FHSCU were asked by the Department of Health to develop a system that would be placed at all FHSAs in England and Wales to enable details of the organs that patients wished to donate to be sent to

UKTSSA. The system operates by setting a number of flags to indicate which organs the patient wishes to donate and holds these against the patient within the FHSA Population Register system. If changes are made to either the patient's administrative details or the patient's organ donor details, then a transaction is automatically generated and passed into the Network for transmission to UKTSSA. UKTSSA will then use that data to update their main database of organ donors.

Therefore the FHSA Population Register could easily be adapted to register patients with a variety of diseases, consideration would have to be given as to how the data would be obtained and kept up to date if this was held at the FHSA Population Register end. If these flags were put against patients on the FHSA Population Register then as well as providing updates to local registers on changes received, the possibility exists that various statistics on large populations could be gathered for use by Public Health within the New Health Authorities. Also it provides the potential for national research to be done by identifying patients to take part in any research trials. In fact on this last point we have already been approached by two researchers, one from Oxford and one from a major hospital in London, to look at providing administrative details on patients from a number of FHSAs around the country for large-scale research projects.

5
Experience Elsewhere in the UK

Overview

This paper reviews how diabetes registers are developing in Scotland.

5.1 Diabetes Registers: A Possible Way Forward in Scotland

Dr Roland Jung, Consultant Physician and Diabetologist, Ninewells
Hospital, Dundee Teaching Hospitals NHS Trust, and Honorary Reader in
Medicine, University of Dundee, Dundee

Introduction

Following a meeting concerning 'the care of diabetic patients in Scotland'
held at the Royal College of Physicians of Edinburgh (RCPEd) in October
1993, a diabetes initiative was established in association with the Scottish
Royal Colleges of Physicians, Scottish Office Home and Health Department,
the Clinical Resource and Audit Group and the Scottish Committee of the
British Diabetic Association with the aim of establishing a plan of action
for the St Vincent Declaration in Scotland. To further this, the Steering
Committee organised sub groups of interested participants to address specific
issues so as to set out the guidelines and quality assurance standards
necessary to meet the St Vincent targets. A further meeting of all concerned
was held at the Royal College of Physicians of Edinburgh in the Autumn of
1994, where each sub group presented their initial report of discussion.
The Steering Committee has before them the reports of all sub groups and
intend to submit these with the final recommendations to the appropriate
bodies in Scotland for discussion.

The following specifically concerns the report of the Task Force on the
topic of Information, Epidemiology and the setting up of Diabetic Registers
in Scotland. This was chaired by Dr R T Jung with representation from a
variety of interested specialties (see Appendix A), which included the
diabetic specialist, the purchaser, public health, epidemiology, nursing,
junior doctor, computer experts, audit and general practice.

Plan for Action

The Task Force considered that the implementation of the general goals
and five year targets embodied in the St Vincent Declaration required
systematic monitoring of the key quality indicators of diabetic care. To
achieve this on a national basis which encompassed each and every diabetic
patient would require the use of information technology and a data set
which ensured quality and completion of retrieval of data. To ensure
completeness of this monitoring, it was considered essential for there to be

set up a *register* of all known diabetic patients with four major components;

a) the register must encompass all known diabetic patients whether followed up or otherwise in the community or in a hospital based setting.

b) The register should be aggregated at the Board/Regional level which then can form part of a national collation.

c) Should be based on the Board of residence of the individual patient. This was considered essential in Scotland, as a person may reside in one area (e.g. North Fife), work in another (e.g. Edinburgh) but attend a Diabetic Centre (e.g. Dundee) in yet a third Board area.

d) The register must be up to date and hence should be updated on an annual basis.

To achieve completeness with quality retrieval of information it was considered essential that the register be based on the *minimum* data necessary for the purposes which would be required from all concerned. Additions to assist with local audit and assessment of local practice would be left to the discretion of those concerned. The group considered that the minimum register must encompass certain demographic information and certain key quality indicators (outcomes or end points) considered *essential* in the St Vincent Declarations. These were as follows;

Demographic

Name; surname, forename
Address
Postcode
Board of residence
Date of birth
Sex
CHI number (or equivalent)

Outcomes

Although the St Vincent Declaration specifically highlights certain goals the definition of the end point was not given in detail and the group therefore consulted widely before stating their definition for the purpose of audit precision. This is best illustrated by 'blindness' where there is no universally accepted definition. In the UK, a person is registered as 'blind' if he or she is unable to perform any work (including social tasks) for which eye sight is essential. In practical terms the degree of visual handicap is understood by this definition to be a visual acuity of <3/60 in the better eye. The WHO has proposed that a person with a visual acuity <6/60 be classified as 'economically blind', whereas those with a visual acuity <3/60 be classified as 'socially blind'. International opinion and EU members favour such re-definition and our report reflected this on going discussion.

It was also essential to measure both prevalence and incidence and to state categorically that every effort should be made to record outcomes solely due to diabetes and not to other causes where possible. An example of this, is again, 'blindness' which in an elderly diabetic patient may be a consequence of senile macular degeneration and not diabetes per se. The outcomes considered essential and their definition were given as follows;

Blindness due to diabetes—prevalence and incidence

Blindness defined as 'registered' blind or eligible for registration with a visual acuity corrected of <3/60 or worse in the better eye; aetiology due to diabetes.

Morbidity from coronary heart disease—prevalence and incidence

1. Onset of angina
2. First myocardial infarct
3. First cardiac revascularisation.

Mortality from coronary heart disease

End stage renal failure due to diabetes—prevalence and incidence

End stage renal failure defined as either a serum creatinine greater than 500 micromoles/l or on dialysis or having received a transplant.

Amputation associated with diabetes—prevalence and incidence

Amputation defined as the first occasion on which a digit or part of a limb was removed other than that as a direct result of trauma.

The register must also include additional data regarding *pregnancy* outcome in female diabetic patients which would include;

live births

maternal mortality consequent of pregnancy

perinatal mortality i.e. stillbirth or death in the first week of life.

termination for congenital malformation
major malformation detected at birth or during the first year of life, i.e. one requiring major surgery or has a major effect on the quality of life of the child.

An important issue necessary for international comparison was that all outcomes should be standardised by the direct method to the European standard population based where appropriate on a 5 year age band. This was also essential for future considered judgmental distribution of resources to improve the quality of care.

The Mechanism of Collection and Analysis

The mechanism of collection of subsequent analysis must be rebust if the data is to be a reliable record. It was considered essential for there to be one person with a contractual responsibility for the activity in each Board (Region), and for Scotland, the most appropriate person was thought to be the Board's Director of Public Health. That person would be responsible for onward transmission of certified accurate data (in the form of tables) to the central collection point for Scotland which the group suggested should be administered by the ISD of the Scottish Health Department. The Royal College of Physicians and General Practitioners would be expected to act in a steering capacity and ensure regular review to update as necessary.

Although the Director of Public Health would have ultimate responsibility of collection and collation, the group did not underestimate the task and recommended the appointment of at least one facilitator for each Board contractually responsible to the Board through the Director of Public Health, and attached to a major local diabetic clinic to re-enforce specialty leadership in diabetes.

The facilitator's role would be as follows;

> To produce the definitive Board register of all diabetic persons resident in that Board's area.

> Liaison with diabetic clinics and general practitioners in other Board areas which have responsibility for follow-up of the Board's patients.

> Responsibility for collecting the yearly returns from all diabetic clinics whether hospital, community or otherwise for the patients on the register, wherever they are attending for follow-up.

> Collation of diabetic pregnancy outcome yearly returns.

> Production of the final outcome tables for onward transmission for national collation.

Data Collection

The method of collection would depend on whether there will be information technology available in the community or hospital involved, the lack of which may be a temporary problem at the outset, for suitable computerisation is *essential* for the long term functioning for such a register.

Hospital Diabetic Clinics have a number of options available;

a) If they already have a computerised register, modification might allow recording and retrieval of the necessary information outlined above. It was considered essential that such databases produce the files necessary to allow transfer of the outcome measures to the facilitator in a form compatible with the proposed system of collation.

b)   The introduction of a basic new database(s) to allow such retrieval.

c)   The introduction of the data set proposed by the British Diabetic Association/Royal College of Physicians (London) working group with specific modification (see Appendix B). This data set was considered extremely comprehensive and would record data far in excess of that required for the St Vincent outcomes, but may be most appropriate to accomplish specific local audit requirements.

d)   For those hospital clinics without any database the group proposed both registration and annual review collation forms as shown in Appendix C. Such would be onward transferred to the facilitator for collation on the outcomes' database.

Once registered the facilitator would send an annual return for each patient for updating as and when seen during the coming year in the clinic. This system was considered possibly also appropriate for the return by certain community practices, particularly where a patient is solely seen at that practice (lead clinician approach).

e)   For the care of children and adolescents the use of existing audit programmes would be suitable if modified to include the essential outcomes as given above.

Community collection posed more difficulties as not all would have the necessary technology and methods to ensure comprehensive collection of data.

To achieve this the group suggested the following method;

a)   To use a 'collection form' (Appendix D) which would be similar to the present community system for retrieving data for such as immunisation. This form would be sent out by the facilitator to each practice detailing their known diabetic patients with recorded end points already known. This form would be returned with the data updated. Newly diagnosed patients would be registered with the facilitator by the practice sending in individual registration forms based on the above 'collection forms'.

Another possibility but as yet untried on a national basis was as follows:

b)   To use the method outlined above (d) for the hospital sector (Appendix C) where registration and annual review form for each individual with diabetes was sent by the facilitator to the practice concerned. This might be most appropriate where a patient is solely seen in the community setting but would require piloting in Scotland to ensure accuracy of retrieval of information, consistency of response and overall acceptability to general practitioners. Difficulty may arise where the practice have their own patient appointment and retrieval system or where there is no lead clinician responsibility for diabetes in each practice. Such systems have worked for thyroid follow-up in Scotland, but this disease requires a far less complex management and audit requirement. Such a system for diabetes is being presently tried out in various English districts using Diabcare, and is the subject of discussion elsewhere.

Shared Care

The collation of data for hospital and community clinics may pose difficulties as regards duplication of patient data and might require to be considered carefully. Obviously the difficulty is most likely to arise when a patient is shared between the hospital and community. We envisage in such circumstance that the facilitator might request retrieval of the hospital data initially then update the practice list before distribution to each individual practice. Such would allow each practice to have a list of their entire diabetic patients where seen alone, shared, or entirely in the hospital service, with the practice updating the list in light of this information.

Finally the facilitator would use an appropriate computer database (to be devised) to produce for the Board the necessary outcome charts, appropriately standardised to the European standard population based where appropriate on 5 year bands.

Finance would be required and was considered necessary as follows;

Capital for hardware and software for facilitator

Revenue for facilitator and overheads

Set-up fee for building a register of all diabetic patients

Review fee for community recall

Capital (and start up revenue) for new hospital based systems (or alteration of existing databases)

Conclusion

The St Vincent Declaration envisages that quality outcomes should be an ongoing process of refinement which might necessitate additions to the proposed data set in due course. Also local audit requirements especially from subspecialty diabetic requirements (e.g. cardiovascular, renal, adolescent, paediatric, pregnancy, foot) would also necessitate specific data sets.

Nevertheless, at the outset, it is necessary to implement retrieval of data to follow those outcomes highlighted as essential goals to assess effective measures for the prevention of complications in the St Vincent Declaration such that *quantity does not drown quality and completeness*. Hence our group emphasised the minimum data retrieval necessary to achieve this purpose.

Appendix A

Appendix A

Membership of the Information and Epidemiology Sub Group for the Implementation of the St Vincent declaration in Scotland.

Dr R T Jung (Chair)	Consultant Physician and Diabetologist, Ninewells Hospital, Dundee Teaching Hospital NHS Trust.
Dr I G Jones	Director of Public Health, Fife Health Board
Professor L Ritchie	Department of General Practice, University of Aberdeen
Dr R Harvey	Senior Registrar in Diabetes, Aberdeen Royal Infirmary
Dr S Siann	Audit Resources and Audit Centre, Kirklands Hospital, Lanarkshire
Miss B Stewart,	Diabetic Nurse Specialists, Crosshouse Hospital, Kilmarnock

Appendix B

Suggested Changes to Dataset

Essential and present

Patient ID	PT_NUM	
Date of record	REC_DATE	
Surname	SURNAME	
Used name	USEDNAME	
Date of Birth	DOB	
Sex	SEX	
Status	DEAD	1=cardiac cause;2=non-cardiac cause;3=moved;4=DNA
Address (1-4)	ADDRESS(1-4)	
Postcode	PC1/PC2	
Year of diagnosis	DIAGNOSIS	Change to year started insulin
Insulin treated	INSULIN	Change to TREAT
Tablet treated	TABLET	Codes: 1=insulin;2=tablet;3=diet
Visual acuity R	VA_R	
Visual acuity L	VA_L	
Serum creatinine	CREAT	
Angina	ANGINA	
MI last year	MI	Change to MI occurred
Amputation leg L	AMPUTLEG_L	Compress to AMPUT_L
Amputation toe/forefoot L	AMPUTOFT_L	Codes: 1=nil;2=above knee;3=below knee;4=forefoot
Amputation leg R	AMPUTLEG_R	Compress to AMPUT_R
Amputation toe/forefoot R	AMPUTOFT_R	Codes: 1=nil;2=above knee;3=below knee;4=forefoot
Background retinopathy L	BACKGND_L	
Preprolif retinopathy L	PREPRO_L	Compress to RETIN_L
Prolif retinopathy L	PROLIF_L	Codes:1=nil;2=diabetic cause;3=non diabetic cause 4=both
Maculopathy L	MACULA_L	
Background retinopathy R	BACKGND_R	
Preprolif retinopathy R	PREPRO_R	Compress to RETIN_R
Prolif retinopathy R	PROLIF_R	Codes:1=nil;2=diabetic cause;3=non diabetic cause 4=both
Maculopathy R	MACULA_R	
Dialysis/transplant	DIALYSIS	Codes: 1=nil;2=current dialysis;3=renal transplant

Essential and absent

Lead clinician	LEAD	
Year of starting insulin	YRINSUL	
Registered blind	REGBLIND	1=nil;2=diabetic cause;3=non-diabetic cause
Year of blind registration	YRBLIND	
Corrected/uncorrected L	CORR_L	
Corrected/uncorrected R	CORR_R	
Date of transplant	TRANSDT	
Year of first amputation	YRAMPUT	
Cause of amputation L	AMPTYP_L	1=diabetic cause;2=non-diabetic cause
Cause of amputation R	AMPTYP_R	1=diabetic cause;2=non-diabetic cause
Year of first angina	YRANGINA	
Year of first MI	YRMI	
CABG done	CABG	
Year of CABG done	YRCABG	
Year of delivery	YRDELIV	
Live birth	LIVE	
Termination of pregnancy	TOP	
Congenital malformation	CONGEN	
Death <1 week	PERI	

Appendix C

Appendix C

REGISTRATION FORM Year ending [31/12/95] Lead Clinician [Dr Gray - Anywhere DGH]

☐ Dead:- cardiac cause   ☐ Dead:- non-cardiac cause   ☐ Moved   ☐ DNA

CHI number [12896785]   D.O.B. [15/3/50]   ☐ Male   ☑ Female

Forename [Jane]   Surname [Smith]

Address [14 Main Street   Carluke   ML8 7HU]

Year of diagnosis [1965]   Current Rx   ☐ Diet   ☐ NIDDM   ☑ IDDM (Started 1965)

Visual acuity   ☐ Registered blind (Date.................)   ☐ Diabetic cause   ☐ Non-diabetic cause

Left   ☐ Not possible   ☐ CF   ☐ PL   ☑ Retinopathy   ☑ Diabetic cause   ☐ Non-diabetic cause
[6/]   Corrected / Uncorrected

Right   ☐ Not possible   ☐ CF   ☐ PL   ☑ Retinopathy   ☑ Diabetic cause   ☐ Non-diabetic cause
[6/]   Corrected / Uncorrected

Renal function

Creatinine [   ]   ☐ Dialysis   ☑ Transplant   (Transplanted 1989)

Lower limb amputations (current status)   Year of first diabetic intervention...

Left   ☐ Above knee   ☐ Below knee   ☐ Forefoot   ☑ Toe   ☐ Diabetic   ☑ Non-diabetic
Right   ☐ Above knee   ☐ Below knee   ☐ Forefoot   ☐ Toe   ☐ Diabetic   ☐ Non-diabetic

---

Ischaemic heart disease

☑ Angina   Onset 1991   ☐ CABG/ Revascularisation   Year of first intervention........................

☐ M.I.   Year of first if known.....................

Pregnancies

	Year of delivery	Live birth	TOP for malformation	Congenital malformation	Perinatal death
1	1974	☑	☐	☐	☐
2	1978	☐	☐	☑	☑
3		☐	☐	☐	☐
4		☐	☐	☐	☐
5		☐	☐	☐	☐

Appendix D

Please complete this form and return as soon as possible to:-

General practitioner:
GP number
GP address:

List of diabetics in area for 19
This lists diabetics on the general practitioner's list on the 31December and those who were diagnosed or transferred onto the list during the calendar year

Diabetics already registered

No.	Date of Birth	CHI No.	Sex	Name and address (including post code)	Pregnant during the year Y/N	Year died	Death due to coronary heart disease (Y/N)	Year[1] became blind due to diabetes	Year developed angina	Year of first myocardial infarction	Year of first cardiac revascularisation	Year[2] developed end stage renal disease due to diabetes	Year[3] of first amputation associated with diabetes

Diabetics not on register

Please add details of diabetics you have diagnosed or treated during the year who are not recorded above

1. Registered blind is <6/60, in the best eye if due to diabetes or registered blind due to diabetes
2. End stage renal disease is defined as a Serum creatinine greater than 500 micromoles/l, on dialysis or having received a transplant due to diabetes.
3. Amputation is defined as the first occasion on which a digit or part of a limb is removed.

Appendix D

Appendix E

TABLE X: Mortality from Coronary Heart Disease in those with Diabetes Mellitus, 19xx, xxxx Health Board

AGE	Number of Those Dying from Coronary Heart Disease During the Year 19xx	
	M	F
15–19		
20–24		
25–29		
30–34		
35–39		
40–44		
45–49		
50–54		
55–59		
60–64		
65–69		
70–74		
75–79		
80–84		
85+		
All Ages		

Bibliography

1   Wilson, A. E., Home P. D. for RCP and BDA. "A data set to allow exchange of information for monitoring continuing diabetic care." *Diabetic Medicine* 10 (1993), 378–390

2   Piwernety, K., Home, P. D., Snogard, O., Antsiferou, M., Staehr-Johansen, K., Krans, M., "Monitoring the targets of the St Vincent Declaration and the implementation of quality management in diabetic care. The Diabcare initiative." *Diabetic Medicine* 10 (1993), 371–377

3   Vaughan, N. J. A. "Measuring the outcome of Diabetes Care." *Diabetic Medicine* 11 (1994), 418–423

4   Jung, R. T., Waugh, N., Scott, A., Chong, P., Browning, M., "A new Pick based computer thyroid register based on the national SAFUR requirements for local usage." *Health Bulletin* 49 (1991), 244–249

5   The care of diabetic patients in Scotland. Prevention of visual impairment and recommended minimum dataset for collection in diabetic patients. A National Clinical Guideline recommended for use in Scotland by the Scottish Intercollegiate Guidelines Network Published March 1996 by SIGN, Royal College of Physicians Edinburgh Publication No 4.